Stresswise

a practical guide for dealing with stress

Dr Terry Looker & Dr Olga Gregson

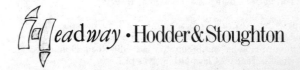

This book is dedicated to our families

British Library Cataloguing in Publication Data

Looker, Terry
  Stresswise: a practical guide for dealing with
  stress.
  1. Man. Stress. Self-treatment
  I. Title II. Gregson, Olga

  ISBN 0 340 50371 8

First published 1989
Reissued 1991

Typeset by Wearside Tradespools, Fulwell, Sunderland
Printed in Great Britain for Hodder and Stoughton Educational, a
division of Hodder and Stoughton Ltd, Mill Road, Dunton Green,
Sevenoaks, Kent by Clays Ltd, St Ives plc.

Contents

Acknowledgements

We are very grateful to Dr Meyer Friedman and the staff of the Recurrent Coronary Prevention Project, Meyer Friedman Institute, San Francisco for providing us with the opportunity to work in the area of stress management.

We also thank our many friends and acquaintances in the United States for their encouragement and time to discuss their work. We would like to express our thanks particularly to Dr Larry Scherwitz and Dr Ray Rosenman.

We thank Vivien Looker for the hours spent deciphering our notes, typing and preparing the manuscript. Also thanks to Taurus Graphics and the Artwork and Illustration Studio for illustrating our work so aptly and to Mike Burge and Holly Gothard of Hodder and Stoughton for their guidance and encouragement throughout the preparation of this book.

From Terry to Vivien, Jodie and Mum and Dad; thank you for your love and support.

Thanks from Olga to Marie, my parents and Jeremy for your steadfast love and support.

Dr Terry Looker graduated from London University in 1969. He lectures and researches in the Department of Biological Sciences at Manchester Polytechnic in the areas of cardiovascular physiology, stress and health. He studied the theory, diagnosis and treatment of Type A behaviour at the Meyer Friedman Institute, San Francisco and established the Coronary-Prone Behaviour Research Unit at Manchester Polytechnic which investigates the relationships between stress, Type A behaviour and heart disease. He developed *Stresswise*, a stress awareness and management programme, and has a private consultancy at Newlands Medical Centre, Bolton. He regularly appears on television and radio and has been featured in articles in professional and technical journals, the national press and popular consumer titles.

Dr Olga Gregson graduated from the University of Wales in 1973. She lectures and researches in the Department of Biological Sciences at Manchester Polytechnic in physiology, behaviour and stress. For the last five years she has had a major interest in stress and health. Together with Dr Looker, she established the Coronary-Prone Behaviour Research Unit. She co-presents *Stresswise*.

Foreword

It is common knowledge that uncontrolled stress can trigger a great many diseases and disorders from insomnia and gastric ulcers, high blood pressure, asthma and migraine to depression and chronic fatigue.

For a long time, however, such problems were treated like something over which we could exercise no control. It was assumed that you could only treat their symptoms with drugs, treat the stress that triggered them off with more drugs, and hope for the best.

Now, thanks to research into altered states of consciousness, deep relaxation, self-awareness and biofeedback, we know that we *can* exercise control over our responses and, once we have gained enough self-awareness and tucked a few stress management skills under our belt, virtually choose how we wish to meet the challenges of our day-to-day lives.

Stress is most assuredly *not* some great dark threat over which we as helpless human beings can exercise little influence. Yet too often in books and articles it is still portrayed that way. In fact, so much nonsense has been written about stress in the industrialised world that it is a pleasure to see *Stresswise* appear in print. Not only does the book avoid the pitfalls of so many of its predecessors – from fuzzymindedness to turgidity to inaccuracy – it also presents a clear, concise and practical account of what stress really is and how to make a friend of it instead of letting it destroy you.

Looker and Gregson are professionals who have done their homework well and know their stuff. But they have other traits in common which endears the book to its reader as well: compassion for instance. They genuinely *care* about life and about helping each and every human being live it to the full. And a sense of humour. They completely avoid the pomposity which too often creeps into books of this kind.

Interesting, thorough and useful, *Stresswise* is a book I can heartily recommend to anyone determined to find out about how to make stress work *for* you rather than *against* you.

Leslie Kenton

Prologue
The Story of Frank

Frank joined a *Stresswise* group counselling course as a last attempt to deal with his emotional problems which had led him to the point of nearly selling his company.

He described his lifestyle and behaviour before joining the course. 'I am very involved in work, have no social activities, get frustrated with employees, have difficulty in delegating and letting someone else do my job, and cannot relax. I am lucky I have an understanding, loving and supportive wife.'

His wife Helen described him as 'totally disorganised, dashing about everywhere and getting nowhere. He is impatient, easily loses his temper over the least thing and does not have much tolerance with anyone. When driving, if a motorist did anything Frank thought he shouldn't have done then Frank made sure the motorist knew about it. He would even stop and hold the traffic up to tell them so. He drives from A to B in the shortest possible time.'

Six months later Frank described how his life had changed as a result of being *Stresswise*. 'I have calmed down considerably and control my temper much better. I drive more slowly and take time off from work to do my own personal things which never happened before. At work I have delegated and left the responsibility to others and sit back and think before making a final decision. I threw my telephone bleep away and started going home earlier and did things around the house. I rearranged my personal commitments that were causing me considerable stress.'

Helen confirmed much of his evaluation. 'He still does not have a lot of tolerance but doesn't fly off the handle at the least thing like he used to. At work he has let people, particularly his foreman, do the job they were employed to do without interfering too much. He is much more content to spend time at home than he ever was. His driving is impeccable, he doesn't exceed

the speed limits or lose his temper with other drivers.'

A year after starting the course, Frank has maintained his new lifestyle. He told the group, 'Since I started the course I have relaxed tremendously; I feel a different person. I was a workaholic when I first came on the course; I couldn't leave work alone. I've just been on holiday for three weeks; the first time in my life I've been away from work for three weeks. When my foreman lost a major contract I did not blow my top, instead I talked it over with him constructively. Since then he has pulled in a lot of work. I do not mind losing contracts if it means I feel the way I do now. You cannot put a price on how I feel now compared to a year ago. I have let go of the reins and let my foreman take the responsibility which I had never been able to do in the past. I make a real effort to get home earlier and do things I never did before such as gardening and preparing the evening meal for Helen when she gets home from work. My driving manner is much better. I drive slower. I see more of life; more of the countryside, I never thought I would get to that stage.'

Frank believes it was his newly gained awareness and understanding of stress that helped him find his own way to deal with it. He knew how stress was affecting him, how he could identify it in himself and how to identify the sorts of things that caused him distress. He was then able to employ the appropriate coping skills to deal effectively with his own situation.

Being *Stresswise* will assist you in doing this. We cannot prescribe a programme of stress management specifically tailored for you as an individual but we can give you the knowledge and practical guidelines so you can decide for yourself what you need to do and how you should go about it.

The Three Sides of Stress

THE GOOD
Excitement, stimulation, creativity, success, achievement, increased productivity.

THE BAD
Boredom, frustration, distress, pressure, poor performance, decreased productivity, failure, headaches, indigestion, colds, unhappy and disharmonious relationships.

THE UGLY
Ulcers, heart attacks, cancer, anxiety, depression, nervous breakdown, suicide.

Introduction

What is Stresswise?

Stresswise is a stress awareness and management programme which tackles stress from its biological roots. It teaches the individual how to develop skills to reduce the bad and undesirable aspects of stress, avoid the ugly, and harness the good and beneficial side of stress. In other words, as the name of the book suggests, this is a practical guide on how to become *wise* about *stress*.

Stresswise is a practical self-help programme. Our aim is to provide an easy-to-follow guide designed to help you deal effectively with stress. This programme was developed from our experience as lecturers and researchers in human stress, performance and health; from studying stress research and management programmes in the United States and from presenting stress awareness and management programmes to a variety of industrial, commercial and professional organisations and individuals from all walks of life.

Another book on stress!

When we approached our publisher with the idea for this book his initial response was 'Another book on stress – how is yours different?'. The first part of this response shows that stress is now an accepted word in our vocabulary even though its precise definition is unclear. It also reflects the growing public concern over the effects of stress on the health of individuals, industry, commerce, the professions and society. In fact, stress has been referred to as 'the twentieth century plague', a description confirmed by the media coverage given to this subject. Hardly a day passes without the appearance of articles in the national press referring to stress. Scanning the newsagent's racks of popular magazines each week will almost certainly reveal features on stress. It is a similar story in professional magazines and journals, particularly business and management titles.

The scale of this attention and coverage originates from the increasing amount of academic research, studies and surveys on stress, health, work and performance. In fact, this research is now so widespread that several new scientific journals have appeared during the last decade to publicise findings. Academic and popular books dealing with stress and stress-related subjects have appeared in increasing numbers during the last twenty years, so why another book on stress and, as our publisher asked, how is *Stresswise* different from other currently available books?

We decided to write *Stresswise* for two reasons. Firstly, the fact that stress is mostly an experience which we create for ourselves means that only we as individuals can control and manage our own stress. Stress management is a skill that can be learned. Although there are many excellent stress and stress management texts currently available, we feel that none provides an educational self-help programme suitable for any individual wishing to learn about stress and how to deal with it.

There are many books aimed at helping specific groups of people such as nurses, executives and managers but what about everyone else? Stress affects everyone. There are many books that deal with specific areas of stress, such as work stress, but ignore other aspects. This may be useful to some degree but stress permeates all aspects of our lives and should therefore be tackled in a holistic manner. So *Stresswise* concentrates on 'self' and our interaction with the environment.

There are also many stress management books containing numerous quotes and references to detailed research, which make it difficult for the reader to extract the key information required to understand the stress concept and to develop effective coping skills. So in writing *Stresswise* we have deliberately avoided using too many quotes and detailed references to scientific studies.

The second reason for putting pen to paper was to satisfy the frequent requests from the participants of our many stress management workshops for a workshop manual to act as a refresher and as a source of reference.

Do you need Stresswise?

Stress is part and parcel of change. Change in our lives means variety. Variety is the spice and sparkle of life. Change also inevitably brings challenges, demands and possible threats. *We can all succeed in living a happier, healthier and more successful life, whatever our current state, if we learn how to handle these demands, challenges and threats more effectively.* To do this we must firstly learn how our bodies respond to stress. We must be able to identify the potential sources of stress and we should learn how stress can affect our health and performance.

Some people seem to cope better with stress than others. This is because we are all different. Our upbringing and personality largely determine our attitudes and expectations. This determines the way we individually deal with the challenges and demands of life. However, we can all benefit from learning more about stress and how to handle it. Admitting to yourself or others that you are suffering from stress is not a sign of weakness. Neither is it a weakness to seek help. Taking lessons to pass the advanced motorist test is not an admission that you are a bad driver but simply that you want to be a better, more effective driver. So in the same way, learning how to manage, handle and cope with stress means you simply want to improve yourself and to be more effective in the things you do.

You would not be alone in feeling that you are suffering from stress. Today, at least three-quarters of those who visit their doctor have a stress-related complaint and many doctors now consider that *almost all* illness and disease is stress-related in some way. Unfortunately, doctors often do not have the time to talk through stress-related disorders with their patients in order to get to the root of the matter. For example, many forms of anxiety and depression are treated with pills and medicines which, whilst necessary and helpful in the short term, cannot solve the underlying problem. Excessive drinking, smoking and drug abuse do not help either. Very often, people are unaware that with appropriate guidance they can go a long way in helping themselves to deal with stress. *Becoming Stresswise is the way to maximise your own natural resources to reduce the bad and avoid the ugly sides of stress and at the same time take advantage of the good side of stress.*

How to use this book

The first part of this book contains a questionnaire from which you will be able to assess the stress in your life and how you behave when you are stressed. To get the most out of this guide, complete the questionnaire before reading Part Two. The questions are designed to direct you into thinking more about stress as it relates to you as you work through Parts Two and Three of the book. Your evaluation of your responses to the questionnaire will help you identify signs, symptoms and sources of stress.

The second part of the book deals with gaining an awareness and understanding of the stress concept. We provide a definition of stress, using a model which we call the 'stress balance'. We look at why stress has become a twentieth century problem. Next, the biology of the stress response is explained so that you are aware of what changes take place in the body when you are stressed. The mental and physical signs of stress are identified and the ways in which stress can lead to ill health and poor performance are described. Finally we look at the sources of stress.

We have found that an understanding of the stress concept is a key factor in bringing about changes in attitude and lifestyle which reduce the undesirable effects of stress and promote its beneficial effects. An understanding of stress is crucial for the effective development of coping skills, which are dealt with in Part Three of the book.

Part Three describes how to deal effectively with stress. It is based on operating the 'stress balance' in order to achieve the right balance. This means altering demands and building up coping resources such as acquiring the ability to relax, learning how not to create unnecessary stress, enhancing self-esteem and the importance of love and support.

At the end of the book you will need to sit back, review your situation and develop your own way of managing stress. To assist you we have provided a *Stresswise* kit containing biodots (small temperature-sensitive devices that can help you learn to relax) together with self-adhesive red hearts and a heart paperclip, to act as stress awareness reminders to help you reduce stressful demands. You will be shown how to use these as you work through Part Three.

This book is a self-help guide and has been written to help everyone. It provides a broad coverage of the subject. Therefore there will inevitably be aspects which are not dealt with in depth or are only mentioned briefly. So for further details and more information, particularly on specific areas such as occupational stress, a list of further reading is given at the end of the book.

We use many examples of situations or events throughout the text to illustrate the subject material. Since *Stresswise* is intended for a diverse readership there may be many instances where, because of differences in the reader's religion, race, social background, marital status, sex and so on, the examples and illustrations may appear to be prejudiced. There is no bias intended and we hope that readers will view any examples used in the widest possible context and apply them as appropriate to their own situation.

Be Stresswise *for health and success*

Wise means knowledgeable. Being *Stresswise* means being knowledgeable about stress so that you can learn the skills to

- reduce your risk of ill health
- enhance your family and social relationships
- improve your performance in the things you do
- increase your productivity and creativity.

Managing stress is ultimately your own responsibility and in your own hands. We hope this book will help you. Good Luck!

PART ONE

*Stress Check
Self-Assessment*

Assess Your Stress

Answer the following questions to find your level of stress. Choose one statement that best describes your response to each question.

1 You are upset by your partner's or colleague's behaviour. Do you

    a Blow up
    b Feel angry but suppress it
    c Feel upset but do not get angry
    d Cry
    e None of the above

2 You must get through a mountain of work in one morning. Do you

    a Work extra hard and complete the lot
    b Forget the work and make yourself a drink
    c Do as much as you can
    d Prioritise the load and complete only the most important tasks
    e Ask someone to help you

3 You overhear a conversation in which a friend/colleague makes some unkind remarks about you. Do you

    a Interrupt the conversation and give him/her a piece of your mind
    b Walk straight by without giving it much thought
    c Walk straight by and think about getting even
    d Walk straight by but sulk about it

4 You are stuck in heavy traffic. Do you

    a Sound your horn
    b Try to drive down a side road to avoid the jam

   c   Switch on the radio or cassette
   d   Sit back and try to relax
   e   Sit back and feel angry
   f   Get on with some work
   g   The question does not apply because you do not have a
       car

5 When you play a sport, do you play to win

   a   Always
   b   Most of the time
   c   Sometimes
   d   Never. I play just for the game

6 When you play a game with children do you deliberately let
   them win

   a   Never. They've got to learn
   b   Sometimes
   c   Most of the time
   d   Always. It is only a game

7 You are working on a project. The deadline is approaching
   fast but the work is not quite right. Do you

   a   Work on it all night and day to make sure it's perfect
   b   Start to panic because you think you will not complete it
       in time
   c   Present your best in the time available without losing
       sleep over it

8 Someone else tidies up your room/office/garage/workshop
   and never places the items/furniture back in the original
   place. Do you

   a   Mark the position of each item and ask the person to put
       it back exactly where it should be
   b   Move everything back to its original position after the
       person has gone
   c   Leave most things as they are – you do not mind the
       occasional shift-round

9 A close friend asks for your opinion about a newly deco-
   rated room. Do you

   a   Think it's awful and say so

b   Think it's awful but say it looks wonderful
c   Think it's awful but comment about the good aspects
d   Think it's awful and suggest improvements

10   When you do something do you

a   Always work to produce a perfect result
b   Do your best and do not worry if it is not perfect
c   Think that everything you do *is* perfect

11   Your family complains that you spend too little time with them because of your work. Do you

a   Worry but feel that you cannot do anything about it
b   Work in the lounge so that you can be with them
c   Take on more work
d   Find that your family has never complained
e   Reorganise your work so that you can be with them more

12   What is your idea of an ideal evening?

a   A large party with lots to drink and eat
b   An evening with your partner doing something you both enjoy
c   Getting away from it all by yourself
d   A small group of friends at dinner
e   An evening with the family doing something you all enjoy
f   Working

13   Which one or more of the following do you do?

a   Bite your nails
b   Feel constantly tired
c   Feel breathless without exertion
d   Drum with your fingers
e   Sweat for no apparent reason
f   Fidget
g   Gesticulate
h   None of the above

14   Which one or more of the following do you suffer from?

a   Headaches

b   Muscle tenseness
c   Constipation
d   Diarrhoea
e   Loss of appetite
f   Increase in appetite
g   None of the above

15   Has one or more of the following happened to you during the last month?

a   Crying or the desire to cry
b   Difficulty in concentrating
c   Forgetting what you were going to say next
d   Little things irritating you
e   Difficulty in making decisions
f   Wanting to scream
g   Feeling that there is no one with whom you can really talk
h   Finding that you are rushing on to another task before you have finished the first one
i   I have not experienced any of the above

16   Have you experienced any of the following during the last year?

a   A serious illness to yourself or someone close to you
b   Problems with your family
c   Financial problems
d   None of the above

17   How many cigarettes do you smoke each day?

a   None
b   One to ten
c   Eleven to twenty
d   Twenty-one or more

18   How much alcohol do you drink a day?

a   None
b   One or two drinks
c   Three to five drinks
d   Six or more drinks

19 How many cups of freshly brewed (not decaffeinated) coffee do you drink a day?

a None
b One or two cups
c Three to five cups
d Six or more cups

20 How old are you?

a 18 or below
b 19–25
c 26–39
d 40–65
e 66 or over

21 You have a very important appointment at 9.30am. Do you

a Have a sleepless night worrying about it
b Sleep well and wake up fairly relaxed but thinking about the appointment
c Sleep well and wake up looking forward to the appointment

22 Someone close to you has died. Of course you are very upset. Do you

a Grieve because no one can ever fill that awful gap
b Grieve because life is so unfair
c Accept what has happened and try to get on with your life

23 You have got into deep water over a problem. Do you

a Reassess the situation by yourself and try to work something else out
b Talk over the problem with your partner or close friend and work something out
c Deny that there is a problem in the hope that the worst may never happen
d Worry about it and do nothing to try and solve it

24 When did you last smile?

a Today
b Yesterday

c   Last week
d   Cannot remember

25   When did you last compliment or praise someone – your children, your partner, colleagues, friends?

a   Today
b   Yesterday
c   Last week
d   Cannot remember

Scores

Add up your score for each question

1   a=0 b=0 c=3 d=0 e=1
2   a=1 b=0 c=1 d=3 e=2
3   a=0 b=3 c=0 d=1
4   a=0 b=0 c=2 d=3 e=0 f=2 g=1
5   a=0 b=1 c=2 d=3
6   a=0 b=1 c=2 d=3
7   a=0 b=0 c=3
8   a=0 b=0 c=3
9   a=0 b=0 c=3 d=1
10   a=0 b=3 c=0
11   a=0 b=0 c=0 d=0 e=3
12   a=1 b=3 c=0 d=1 e=2 f=0
13   a=0 b=0 c=0 d=0 e=0 f=0 g=0 h=1
14   a=0 b=0 c=0 d=0 e=0 f=0 g=1
15   a=0 b=0 c=0 d=0 e=0 f=0 g=0 h=0 i=1
16   a=0 b=0 c=0 d=2
17   a=3 b=1 c=0 d=0
18   a=3 b=2 c=1 d=0
19   a=3 b=2 c=1 d=0
20   a=0 b=0 c=1 d=2 e=3
21   a=0 b=1 c=3
22   a=0 b=0 c=3
23   a=2 b=3 c=0 d=0
24   a=3 b=2 c=1 d=0
25   a=3 b=2 c=1 d=0

Your score

51–68: Your stress level is low. You show very few signs of stress. You are not a workaholic. You show Type B behaviour and cope very well with stress generally.

33–50: Your stress level is moderate. You show some stress. You are not a workaholic but there is some tendency for it. You show mild Type A behaviour and generally cope quite well with stress.

16–32: Your stress level is high. You show many signs of stress. It is likely that you are a workaholic. You display moderate Type A behaviour and do not handle stress very well.

0–15: Your stress level is very high. You show a great deal of stress. You are a workaholic. You display extreme Type A behaviour and your ability to deal with stress is very poor.

Your stress level scores are based on some of the main themes developed in this book. Bear in mind your score and these factors as you progress through the guide:

- Signs of stress
- Type A behaviour
- Attitude to work
- Attitude to life
- Lifestyle

PART TWO

*Awareness of
the Stress Concept*

Just as a car can be serviced and tuned for peak performance and to avoid or reduce problems and breakdowns, so too can our bodies be prepared to run smoothly and perform well. Such self servicing includes learning the skills to deal with stress effectively so as to avoid the ugly side of stress, reduce the bad and promote the good. An essential step in this process is to gain an awareness and understanding of the stress concept. This is what this part of the book is about.

To tune a car you must know how it works and be able to recognise the symptoms of both a poorly tuned and a properly running engine. Tuning your ability to deal with stress means understanding what stress is, how it affects the body and how to recognise the signs and symptoms of stress.

Once you have gained this knowledge you must then acquire the tools to carry out the necessary adjustments. You can learn the skills to review, adjust and tune your behaviour, attitude and lifestyle in Part Three of the book.

1 Stress: A Twentieth Century Problem?

Stress affects everyone. It is a necessary and essential part of our lives, an inevitable result of the interaction between us and our environment. We need stress to be able to adapt to the continual changes of our environment and to keep us on our toes in order to survive.

One way of looking at stress is to regard it as an adaptive response by the body to changes in the environment. The stress response evolved to enable man to deal with life-threatening dangers, for example being confronted by a predator such as a sabre-toothed tiger. Activation of this stress response very quickly prepared the body for physical activity: to stand and fight or turn tail and flee. This was obviously a necessary action for the survival of our cave-dwelling ancestors. For early man in his harsh and inhospitable environment, threats and demands were predominantly physical. Satisfying life support needs was a struggle: hunting for food, keeping warm and finding shelter probably took most of his time and energy.

Today, in our advanced technological and computerised world, we live in a 'convenience' society. How easy life is – tonight's dinner is enticingly packaged on the hypermarket shelves with a choice and variety undreamt of even 20 years ago. We have no physically demanding hunting trip, instead we just jump into the car and drive to the store, park, walk in, pick up the meal, pay and drive home. Cooking is simply turning a switch on the cooker or microwave; no strenuous gathering and chopping of wood and then making a fire. We sit down at the dining table in the comfort of a centrally heated house; no need to look over our shoulder for danger while we eat – the lurking sabre-toothed tiger or a raiding party from another tribe are not there. How different it is today, or is it?

Let us take the above illustration and re-examine it; the scene is probably more along the following lines. We get into the car and drive to the shops but on the way we have to pick up the children from school, collect the dog from the vet and do a whole list of other jobs, only to find that the car will not start or we get caught in a traffic jam or we get a flat tyre. Arriving at the shopping centre we search for a parking space then once in the shops we get pushed and jostled by the crowds. At the checkout we queue impatiently only to realise as we are about to pay that we have left our purse or wallet at home. Then the electric fuse blows as we are cooking . . .

These examples illustrate the kinds of demanding situations that each of us faces at some time. Not only can we feel physically threatened, we can also feel psychologically threatened, by threats to our self-esteem, our security, our role in society and our relationships with family, friends and fellow humans. We live in a world where the rate of change and the type of changes we face have dramatically increased and continue to do so. The queue at the supermarket checkout and the traffic jam can become the fangs of the sabre-toothed tiger and when confronted by these threats we respond just as if that tiger were there – by activating our caveman stress response. Having activated our body for an immediate physical response, there is often no need or no opportunity for any physical action! We cannot hurry the queue in the supermarket or the traffic jam. We cannot fight the queue; we cannot run away from it either. So we become impatient and irritated; we become angry; we fume!

Because of the structure of western society most of our time is spent in complex and often confusing social interaction. This interaction has become very complicated because of the effects of urbanisation and the types of society we have created since our cave-dwelling days. Competition appears more evident today than ever before: competing for jobs, striving for career promotion. Sadly, in today's society we tend to get caught up in the 'rat race'. We become pulled along in a tide of emotional and social demands and at the same time we have to find work and earn a living or face redundancy and unemployment. So inevitably our stress response is activated whether it is warranted or not. Often we can find ourselves in a state of high alertness but without the appropriate outlets for physical expression. Our body may become prepared for a fight if we see the boss as the sabre-toothed tiger, lurking behind his desk, threatening our self-esteem, career prospects or job security, but we cannot leap into physical action. We may feel angry and aggressive but cannot hit out or engage in physical conflict. Instead we fume inside, hit the bottle or vent our anger on others – often our loved ones.

This is where many researchers and doctors believe part of the trouble lies; *activation of our stress response without the physical activity that is meant to follow can be potentially harmful to health.*

Threats to our self-esteem and the security of our relationships and jobs are the result of an increasingly changing society. So rapid have been these changes that our bodies and our biology have simply not had time to keep pace. Again it is here that our problem lies. *We are dealing with today's social demands by using a stress response designed to allow our ancestors to deal with physical dangers.* Today, the threat of losing a job, the struggle and fight to reach the top of the career ladder, the struggle to find employment, job stress, marital and family disharmony, loneliness and financial problems are some situations that can gnaw away at us over a long period. This means that our body defences are in a constant state of activation, albeit of varying degrees, in resisting these threats and demands. This can also lead to ill health and in certain cases, death. It is ironic that the very system developed to protect us can be today's number one killer!

So it is not stress in itself that is a twentieth century problem. The increased intensity, number, frequency, pattern and variety of demands placed on the body activates the stress response in such a way that may ultimately become detrimental to health – *this* is a twentieth century problem! So what *is* stress?

2   What is Stress?

Stress can be good, bad and ugly

When asked to define stress, most people usually refer to its bad
side. They describe stress as an unpleasant experience, for
example being under too much or too little pressure, feeling
frustrated or bored, being in situations which they feel unable to
handle or control, thinking that they are a failure, experiencing
marital disharmony, bereavement or financial difficulties. What
they are in fact describing is DISTRESS – the *bad* aspect of stress.
This, left unchecked, can lead to poor performance, decreased
productivity and ill health. For the individual, distress can give
rise amongst other things to headaches, indigestion, frequent
colds, neck and back ache and unhappy relationships. For the
company and organisation, distress is seen in terms of absenteeism, lost production, poor work performance, accidents, reduced creativity and lack of innovation. Distress can also be
ugly. This is the more extreme form of bad stress, leading to
physical disability or even death as a result of heart attacks,
cancer, anxiety, depression and nervous breakdown.

On the other hand, some people describe stress as a pleasant,
exciting, stimulating and thrilling experience. They feel completely capable of handling the demands they face and deliberately put themselves into challenging situations which they
know they can handle. The stress they are experiencing is called
EUSTRESS – or *good* stress. Tackling interesting and stimulating
tasks, being creative and productive, achieving goals and de-
sires, participating in competitive sports can be the joys of
stress. Here stress is working for us to improve our performance.

Stress is an experience which is unique to each and every one
of us. What is distressful for one individual can be positively
eustressful for another person. Deliberately putting ourselves
into challenging situations can be distressful as well as eustressful. Someone about to take his first parachute jump may be

overcome with fear and unable to jump (distress). An experienced parachutist will jump without worrying about the potentially life-threatening situation and enjoy the thrill of the jump but with the stress response in a high state of arousal he will be alert and ready to deal with any problems that may arise (eustress).

In this example the situation or demand, the jump, is the same for both parachutists but each experiences a different feeling and level of stress. This is because each assesses the nature of the demand and his own ability to cope with it.

A definition of stress

Stress can therefore be defined as a state we experience when there is

> *a mismatch between perceived demands and perceived ability to cope. It is the balance between how we view demands and how we think we can cope with those demands that determines whether we feel no stress, distressed or eustressed.*

This can be illustrated and explained by using a simplified model which we have called the stress balance (Figure 1). It is

Perceived demands (D)   Perceived coping
                               resources/ability (C)

Fig. 1   The stress balance

important that you study this model carefully as it forms the basis of this guide to stress management. We will refer to it throughout the book.

The stress balance

In the pan on one side of the balance are what we see as the demands (shown as D) around us. In the other pan is what we see as our ability to cope or deal with those demands (shown as C). When we feel able to handle our demands then C will balance D. This does not mean, however, that the scales are necessarily perfectly horizontal. Because we are dealing with a psychological phenomenon, we do not know how much of C is needed to be in total balance with D. We do not necessarily have to have equal weights in each pan in order to be in balance. Rather, the scales should be seen as fluctuating up and down to some degree through a 'zone' of balance, which we will refer to as the 'normal zone' (Figure 2). The extent of this zone will be different for every individual and indicates that the body is operating in a normal and healthy way. In this zone we would not say we are experiencing stress. The normal zone can be regarded as our everyday living zone, or normal situations zone,

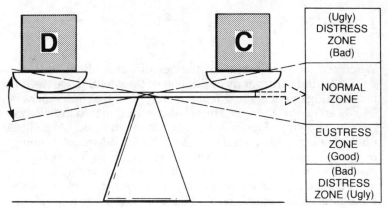

Situation: fluctuations in perceived demands and perceived coping resources but balance remains in the normal stress zone.

Fig. 2   The normal zone

in which we are dealing with familiar and routine daily changes in our environment and with everyday demands that, through our experience, we know pose no major threats. Our body adapts to the changing situation by activating our stress response to a degree that we are hardly aware of. In fact, if we were fully conscious of every little change in our body, we would be less effective in dealing with challenges, novel and emergency situations when these arise. So the stress response is always in a low state of activity; held in a state of readiness for further or full activation but without us constantly experiencing stress.

Of course there will be times when small changes in D and C will occur, perhaps as a result of inevitable daily hassles and not feeling too well, so the balance will tip one way and then the other. As long as these fluctuations are within the normal zone of balance then we would not say we are distressed or eustressed but perhaps we would say we felt a little niggled or stimulated at times. It is when the balance tips outside the normal zone that we experience stress as distress or eustress and clearly the more imbalance the stronger these feelings will be. Imbalance can occur in two ways:

1   alterations in perceived nature of demands
2   changes in perceived ability to cope.

Distress

When we face an increased number of demands or view the demands that confront us as difficult or threatening, we need to make a judgement about our ability to cope. If that judgement is, 'No, I can't cope' then the stress balance can tip into the distress zone as shown in Figure 3. Having too much to do in too little time; dealing with complex tasks without adequate training; promoted into a job for which we are not suited; having too many bills to pay and not enough income; worrying how we will manage if we lose our job; having domestic problems at the same time as changes at work. These are just a few examples of the kinds of demands that can lead to distress. Of course, the list could be endless and being *Stresswise* will help you identify those situations which put *you* in the distress zone.

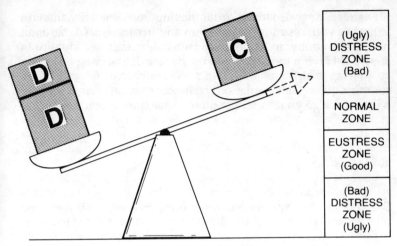

Situation: perceived ability to cope with increased demands
does not match – distress is experienced.

Fig. 3   The distress zone I

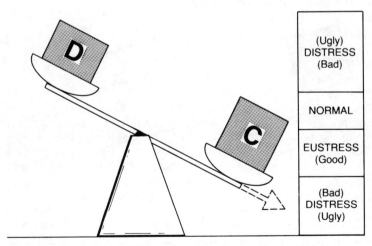

Situation: perceived ability to cope far outweighs the perceived
demands; boredom, frustration – distress experienced.

Fig. 4   The distress zone II

Distress can also arise from having too few demands to stimulate you, resulting in boredom and frustration. In this case, perceived ability to cope outweighs demands as shown in Figure 4. Having too little to do or too few demanding tasks can be just as distressful as having too much to do or tackling complex jobs. This situation commonly arises when people retire or are given jobs which do not match their abilities.

Eustress

Eustress can be experienced when our perceived ability to cope outweighs our perceived demands as shown in Figure 5. Although we have an imbalance here, clearly this is a desirable one. In this respect eustress can be regarded as an extension of the normal zone of the stress balance.

Notice here that this situation is different from that described in Figure 4 where distress results from having too few demands. The eustress situation gives rise to a feeling of confidence, of being in control and able to tackle and handle tasks, challenges and demands. The stress response is activated by just the right

Situation: perceived ability to cope outweighs the perceived demands; confident and in control – eustress experienced.

Fig. 5   The eustress zone

amount to provide the alertness, the mental and physical performance required to be productive and creative.

Getting the balance

Because of the way we live today, we are almost certain to feel distressed at some time or another so we need to reduce the frequency and extent to which the stress balance tips into the distress zones. We can do this by decreasing the number and types of demands and by building up our coping resources. This will help to avoid or to minimise the effects of distressful situations. We need to learn how to increase our excursions into the eustress zone by getting the *right* balance between demands and coping resources. *To get the right balance we need to reappraise how we perceive and interact with our environment* because this determines the way we match up our demands with our ability to cope.

Now that the terms 'distress' and 'eustress' have been introduced and defined, these will be used throughout the book. When the term 'stress' alone is used this will refer to any degree of activation of the stress response outside the normal zone; that is, both distress and eustress. The activity of the stress response in the normal zone should be considered as an inevitable part of our lives and when in this zone we do not experience 'stress'.

We cannot live a life devoid of distress so the important thing is not to allow our stress balance to remain in the distress zone and not to stray into this zone too far and too often. Instead we should aim to use our stress response to improve our lives and performance by keeping our balance in the normal and eustress zones. This can be achieved by learning the skills to alter the balance between demands and coping ability and this is the basis for the effective stress management dealt with in Part Three. In order to learn these skills it is necessary to understand how the stress response operates in the body, what it does and how to recognise the signs and symptoms of distress and eustress.

3 The Stress Response

Why you need to learn about the stress response

Almost everyone we have taught and counselled agrees that gaining an awareness and understanding of the stress response is an important and necessary step in the bid to deal effectively with stress. You need to learn about the biology of the stress response if you are to understand and appreciate how to recognise the signs and symptoms of stress, how stress can lead to health problems and affect performance, and the way in which stress can arise through the way we behave. More importantly, you will know something about the biological reasons for carrying out the coping exercises we describe in Part Three, and you will also appreciate why these coping strategies have been adopted.

NB: What follows is a very simplified general account of a complex response, much of which is not yet fully understood. We advise you to read this chapter carefully.

What is the stress response?

The term 'stress response' describes a series of different and complex responses made by the body to any demand it faces. The stress response is always active to some degree, operating within the normal zone of the stress balance to enable us to deal with everyday changes in the environment. When unusual, novel or excessive demands, challenges or threats arise, the stress response ensures that the body is always in a state of readiness to deal with them. Because demands can be life-threatening, physical, emotional, pleasant or unpleasant, the body's response must be appropriate for dealing with the type of situation faced. It would not be effective and economical for the body to activate a single fixed stress response to deal with all eventualities, so different parts and levels of the stress response are activated to enable us to respond in the most appropriate way.

If we are suddenly confronted by an actual life-threatening situation such as a car hurtling out of control towards us or someone about to attack us, our response must be immediate. The body goes on an emergency full alert and prepares for physical activity. Because of the speed and urgency of this level of response it has been called the **alarm reaction** and also the **emergency response**. It may be that running away from danger will preserve our life or it could be that staying to fight will be more effective. We decide in a fraction of a second which course of action to take.

The alarm reaction evolved to prepare our cave-dwelling ancestors for action when confronted by a wild animal or similar threat. A split-second decision had to be made on whether to stand their ground and fight or turn tail and flee as fast as possible. So another name for the alarm reaction is the **fight or flight response**.

The alarm response is not an appropriate way to deal with long-term threats and demands. Here we need to make continual adjustments over a relatively long period of time. This mainly involves another part of the stress response called the **resistance reaction**.

Many of the demands we face today are not necessarily directly life-threatening (life or death situations) but nevertheless pose threats and challenges to our personal security and well-being. These demands are usually emotional rather than physical in nature. Some arise unexpectedly and suddenly and last only a short time whilst others persist for a long period; gnawing away day after day, week after week and even year after year. These long-term demands may include maintaining and protecting our own and our family's well-being and relationships, finding and keeping a job or earning a living and striving for promotion. Dealing with these situations is often distressful since it can involve struggling to establish control or fearing that control might be lost and, as a result, the safety and well-being of self and family is threatened.

How then is it decided which part of the stress response is

activated so that the body can deal appropriately with the situation it faces?

Activation of the appropriate part of the stress response is the result of our assessment of the situation and how we think we can deal with it. This interpretation process then sets into motion a physiological reaction by the body to produce the right type of stress response. It is important to distinguish here between situations that are sudden, life-threatening ones, such as jumping clear of a car, and those which pose no actual physical threat to our life, such as being interviewed for promotion at work. For sudden, life-threatening situations there is an immediate and total activation of all parts of the stress response. However, for situations which are more psychological or emotional in nature, the stress response is activated to an appropriate degree to enable us to deal effectively with the demands we face. In this book we are dealing mainly with the latter category.

Another point to remember is that *any* expression of the stress response is based on either the alarm (fight or flight) response or the resistance response, or both. For example, the alarm response is usually triggered just enough to allow us to deal with immediate and short-acting demands which are not life-threatening, so we may experience a little aggression or a little fear. However, sometimes we may feel so emotionally threatened by a situation (whether or not it is warranted) that the alarm response is activated to such a level that we become quite aggressive – we decide to mentally 'fight' and our body is prepared for fighting. This is one way of coping with the situation.

On the other hand we may feel that the demand is too much for us to handle so we become scared – we mentally 'run away' from the situation while at the same time our body is geared for flight. Our emotions, for example fear or anger, therefore play a major part in our interpretation and assessment of the situation we face and hence the degree and pattern of activation of our stress response.

Basically we can interpret a situation in three ways:

'I can cope with this situation' – perceived coping ability outweighs perceived demands.
'I am not sure whether I can cope with this situation' – doubt about perceived ability to cope with perceived demands.
'I cannot cope with this situation' – perceived demands outweigh perceived coping ability.

If we feel that we can handle the situation, the stress response is activated within the normal zone of the stress balance and we do not feel stressed. If we are uncertain about coping or if we feel unable to cope with a demand, the stress response will be activated beyond its normal zone giving rise to varying degrees of distress and accompanying mental 'fight or flight' or 'resistance' reactions. When we feel confident that we can deal with a demand, the stress response goes into the eustress zone. In this case we often look forward to the challenge that a situation presents and as a result we experience eustress.

The differences in the extent of activation of the stress response within or beyond the normal zone of the stress balance depend on how you view or interpret situations around you and on how you feel about those situations. This means that stress is not in the environment but is a *state within you*. The way in which you interact with the environment determines how much and what type of stress you create for yourself.

> *'Men are disturbed not by things but by the views which they take of them.'* Epictetus

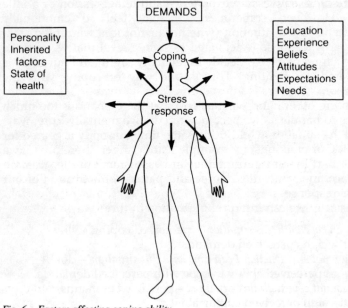

Fig. 6   Factors affecting coping ability

Our interpretation of the nature of the demand and how well we feel able to cope with it depends on our experience of past events, our beliefs, attitudes, expectations and needs. These in turn depend on our genetic inheritance, personality, education, upbringing, age, sex and general state of health (Figure 6).

So, bearing in mind the interpretative processes going on, we can now relate how we view the situation to how the body responds physiologically to produce the appropriate level and type of stress response activation.

The appropriate response is ultimately achieved by altering the activity of the body organs to prepare the body for action. It is the job of particular chemical messengers in the body to alter organ activity. Different messengers produce different effects; for instance, one particular messenger speeds up the heart beat, while another messenger may effect a decrease in heart rate.

The type and amount of messenger required for a particular task is decided by the brain after it has received information from the senses about the nature of the demand:

'Is it life threatening?'
'Does it need to be dealt with immediately or can it wait?'

The brain also assesses how we feel about the situation:

'Can I face up to it?'
'Am I in control of the situation?'
'I am angry about this.'
'I am concerned about this.'

The brain also recalls information from its memory store about what was learned in previous encounters.

'What did I do in this situation before?'
'This is a new experience, I'll have to tread carefully with this one.'

All these pieces of information are taken into consideration for a decision on the most appropriate course of action. Once a decision has been reached it is transmitted to part of the brain called the **hypothalamus** which sets into motion the various chemical messengers required to bring about a response by the body.

It really is an issue of

'ON YOUR MARKS' – *'Here is a demand I have to deal with'*
Brain collects information, processes it, assesses the situation and decides on a course of action.

'GET SET' – *Preparing to deal with the demand*
Brain (hypothalamus) activates stress response to a degree relative to the interpreted nature and importance of the demand.

'GO' – *Dealing with the demand*
Type of resulting action depends on interpretation of situation and emotions.

Let us take two situations and examine them in terms of what is happening within the categories of 'On your marks', 'Get set', 'Go'.

Example 1: Potential life or death situation. Confrontation by a bull about to charge.

ON YOUR MARKS

'Here is a demand I have to deal with'
'I see the bull. It looks threatening. I must get away quickly.'

GET SET

Preparing to deal with the demand
Body preparing to run.

GO

Dealing with the demand
Run away as fast as possible. Full activation of the stress response. Heart beats harder and faster. Breathing more rapid and deeper. Energy stores mobilised. Blood directed to muscles. Muscles contract for action.

Example 2: Non life or death situation. Job interview, which is not going too well. Emotionally, the interviewee sees the situation as fearful, and feels unable to cope. The stress response is activated to a degree that tips the stress balance beyond the normal zone, resulting in distress. The stress response is expressed in the 'flight' mode.

ON YOUR MARKS

'Here is a demand I have to deal with'
'I am not doing very well in this interview. I haven't answered the questions well and I've made a fool of myself. I wish I could get out of here as quickly as possible.'

GET SET

Preparing to deal with the demand
Body preparing to run but cannot actually run away.

GO

Dealing with the demand
Mentally running away but physically having to stay and face the situation. Heart beats harder and faster. Breathing rapid and shallow. Muscles tensed ready for action. Blood directed to muscles away from gut. Stomach feels as though it is twisting and churning.

Example 1 illustrates the activation of the stress response in terms of the flight aspect of the alarm reaction. The life or death situation, such as facing a charging bull, requires full activation of the stress response, directed toward the flight part of the alarm response to increase chances of survival. In this case the stress response is being used for the purpose for which it was evolved. Running away will hopefully save our life. Each and every one of us has this response. It is there to help us survive.

However, the very same response is triggered when we feel like running away in a non life or death situation, such as that in example 2 where the interview is not going our way. Here the stress response is not activated to its fullest extent because we are not dealing with a life or death situation. In this case the body is prepared physically to run away but this is not possible. We usually have to stay and face the situation. The desire to flee without the opportunity to do so produces a very different body reaction to actually running away.

It must be emphasised that all our responses to non life-threatening situations are simply varying degrees of activation of our alarm (fight or flight) or resistance responses, or both of these. The problem in today's society is that in non life-threatening situations the stress response is often almost as extreme as if the situation were physically threatening. We therefore need to learn to handle non life-threatening situations so as not to tip the stress balance into the distress zone. Being *Stresswise* will achieve this.

In example 2, for instance, the interviewee feels things are not going very well. He perceives that the demands of the interview now outweigh his ability to cope with the situation, the balance tips out of the normal zone and he will feel distressed. The more the demands outweigh the ability to cope, the more the stress response is activated and in this particular case the more the flight aspect of the stress response is manifested in the interviewee's body actions. Here, the interviewee interpreted the situation as one which he would like to escape from and the body is prepared to do so.

These examples illustrate how the expression of our stress response can be related to our interpretation of the situation and to our emotional state. Although we know that our emotions do affect the expression of the stress response, the present state of knowledge of this link is limited. For example, depending on the individual and on the situation, a person's different emotional states such as anxiety, anger, fear, happiness, or no emotion at all, can result in one and the same level of stress response activation.

We now need to explain what actually happens in the body during the ON YOUR MARKS, GET SET, GO sequence. You will then be able to identify the signs of your stress response and consequently discover the sources of your stress and how stress can affect your health and performance. You will also appreciate the basis behind the coping strategies and skills that are dealt with in Part Three. So take a little extra time to study this next section.

ON YOUR MARKS

'Here is a demand I have to deal with'

Our senses pick up information about our environment and pass this to the brain for processing, interpretation and decision-making. We are on standby, ready to deal with danger, threats and demands. A demand arises, our brain assesses the situation and establishes how we can best deal with that demand. If we feel that we can cope, the stress response is activated to an appropriate degree and operates within the normal zone of balance. Activation of the stress response beyond its normal zone will occur only when it is judged that the demand cannot be handled (distress) or that it can be easily and confidently dealt with (eustress) as we have discussed above.

Having assessed the situation, our body must prepare for the appropriate action.

GET SET

Preparing to deal with the demand

Once the brain has decided on a course of action, the 'get set' instructions are passed to the body organs, leading to an attempt by the body to deal with the situation. It may be that the decision, based on our interpretation of the situation and our emotions, is appropriate and our response is successful in dealing with the demands. In this case we will feel no distress, and may experience eustress.

However, it may be that the decision is inappropriate or our response to the situation is ineffective, in which case we will experience distress.

So how are the 'get set' instructions passed to the body to bring about a response to the situation faced?

The brain–body action link

Instructions from the brain to the body are carried in the form of small electrical impulses which are sent along nerves directly from the brain to the body organs. When these impulses arrive at the end of the nerve, small amounts of a chemical (called a **neurotransmitter**) are released onto the cells that make up the

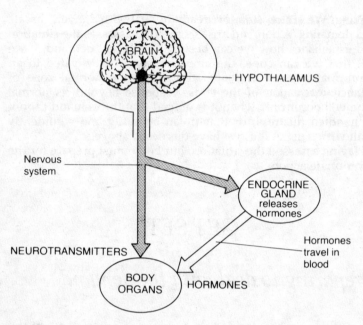

Fig. 7   The brain-body link

organ. The neurotransmitter alters the activity of the organ.
Another way in which messages reach the organs is by a special
chemical messenger, called a **hormone**. This is released from
special glands (**endocrine glands**) and travels in the blood to the
organs. Hormones also alter the activity of the organs enabling
the body to prepare for action (see Figure 7).

Several neurotransmitters and hormones are released to initiate the stress response and each triggers a different set of
actions by the organs. *It is the different patterns of body organ
activity that result in either alarm response initiation, resistance
response initiation or varying degrees of activation of both responses
together.*

The brain works out the most appropriate pattern of body
activity to deal with the demand, and then sets into motion a
sequence of events leading to the release of the appropriate
cocktail of neurotransmitters and hormones to achieve this
response. To understand how this happens you will need to
learn a little about the brain and the links with the body organs
via the nervous and hormone systems.

'Get set' instructions from the brain via the nervous system

The nervous system is made up of about a billion nerve cells called **neurones**. Each neurone is connected to many hundreds of other neurones to form a complex communication system along which electrical **nerve impulses** are sent. Nerve impulses are the language of the nervous system and the means by which the brain communicates with the body organs.

You will see in Figure 8 that the neurone endings do not have physical contact with the body organ. There is a minute gap between them so the message is carried by the neurotransmitter over the gap to the body organ. The neurotransmitter is stored in small packets inside the neurone endings. When an electrical impulse arrives at the neurone ending the packets burst open releasing the chemical onto the surface of the body organ. When the cells of the body organ receive the neurotransmitter message the activity of that organ is altered.

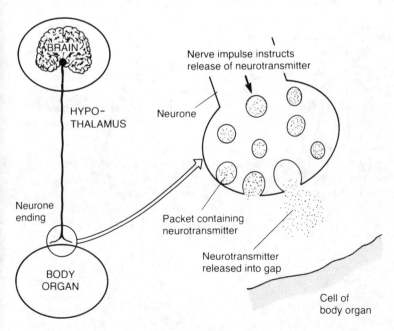

Fig. 8   Communication between neurone ending and cell of body organ

The two parts of the nervous system

We have a conscious or voluntary control over some parts of the body, including the muscles of the limbs and body wall. We can consciously instruct our arm or leg to move at will. The nerves from the brain to these organs form a part of our nervous system called the **voluntary nervous system** (Figure 9). On the other hand we have very limited conscious control over the activity of the body organs (heart, stomach, lungs, glands and blood vessels). These areas of the body are controlled by the other part of our nervous system called the **autonomic nervous system**. This system works automatically to ensure that vital body processes such as the heart beating, breathing and digestion do not stop and are adjusted to deal with changing conditions. For instance, the rate of beating of the heart is altered automatically to ensure that the right amount of blood is delivered to the muscles of the arms and legs depending on their level of activity – the harder they work, the more blood is required. The autonomic nervous system is involved in the everyday running and maintenance of the body's normal activities and is operat-

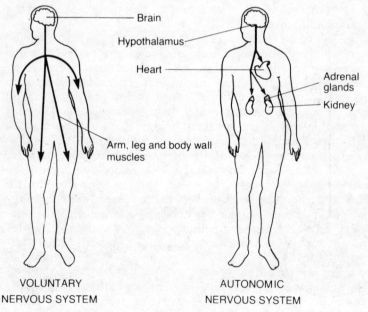

Fig. 9   Voluntary and autonomic nervous systems

ing continuously 24 hours a day, 7 days a week, every moment of our lives.

The autonomic nervous system is of most interest to us in understanding how the stress response is activated, since *changes in the level of autonomic nervous system activity produce the body actions necessary for dealing with demands.*

When the stress response is operating within the normal zone, autonomic nervous system activity will maintain normal functions and enable us to deal with common everyday demands. Full activation of the stress response involves the highest level of autonomic nervous system activity. Where the event is not life-threatening the stress response is activated enough to deal with the demand and this is brought about by an appropriate change in activity of the autonomic nervous system. It is the interpretation of the demand that will ultimately determine the extent of activity in the autonomic nervous system and hence activation of the stress response.

The autonomic nervous system is actually two separate systems: the **sympathetic nervous system** and the **parasympathetic nervous system**. It is mostly through increased sympathetic activity that the stress response is activated. The parasympathetic nervous system also has a role to play here because of the corresponding decrease in its activity.

The role of the parasympathetic nervous system is to conserve energy, to aid digestion and to defend the body from the invasion of foreign material such as bacteria. Increasing activity in the parasympathetic nervous system results, for example, in increased secretion of the eyes (tears), mouth (saliva), nose and lungs (mucus) and stomach (acid gastric juice). These secretions trap and destroy foreign material (Figure 10).

On the other hand the main role of the sympathetic nervous system is to expend energy. The body is prepared for action, for exercise and to deal with emergency situations by initiating the alarm response. Increasing sympathetic activity results, for example, in an increase in the heart rate, more blood flow to the muscles and quicker and deeper breathing (Figure 10).

The action of the sympathetic nervous system is largely brought about by a neurotransmitter called **noradrenaline**. Parasympathetic action is mainly brought about by a neurotransmitter called **acetylcholine**.

Most body organs receive messages from both divisions of the autonomic nervous system. However, there are some which receive messages from only one of the branches. For example,

Fig. 10   Summary of autonomic nervous system activity

the adrenal medulla, spleen and sweat glands receive messages from the sympathetic division only, whilst some of the salivary glands receive only a parasympathetic supply. *This pattern of nerve supply distribution is important in determining body organ activity and allows a variety of different responses to be made by the body depending on the circumstances.*

The table opposite shows the effects on body organ activity of stimulating the parasympathetic and sympathetic nerves.

You will notice that sympathetic stimulation causes increased activity in some organs, for example heart muscle, but reduced activity in others, such as gut muscles. Similarly, parasympathetic stimulation increases activity in some organs, such as gut muscles, but decreases activity in others, for example heart muscle. Where an organ has both sympathetic and parasympathetic nerve supplies, sympathetic stimulation increases the activity whereas parasympathetic stimulation decreases activity. For example, an increase in sympathetic activity while parasympathetic activity is low will result in a higher heart rate than normal. This is what happens if we increase our level of muscular activity, for example in exercising. On the other hand an increase in parasympathetic activity while sympathetic activity is low will result in a lower heart rate and this happens when we are rested and relaxing.

ORGAN/TISSUE	PARASYMPA-THETIC EFFECT	SYMPATHETIC EFFECT
Heart	Decreased rate	Increased rate and force of beat
Blood vessels	Generally little or no effect but can cause dilation (widening) of blood vessels to heart muscle, lungs, brain and sex organs	Constrict except those supplying heart muscles, leg and arm muscles which dilate
Spleen	−	Contracts and empties stored red blood cells into the circulation
Salivary glands	Increased flow of saliva	Decreased flow of saliva
Gut muscles	Increased movement	Decreased movement
Lung airways	Constrict, decreasing air flow	Dilate, increasing air flow
Sweat glands	−	Increased sweating
Pupils of eye	Contraction of sphincter muscle; pupil becomes smaller − constricts	Contraction of radial muscle of iris; pupil becomes wider − dilates
Liver and fat tissue	−	Mobilisation of sugar and fat
Brain, mental activity	−	Mental activity increased
Blood	−	Increased ability to clot

(−) = Little or no effect

Most organs of the body have a dominant control by either the sympathetic or parasympathetic systems. For example, the heart and blood vessels are controlled predominantly by the sympathetic nervous system.

Blood flow throughout the body is regulated almost entirely by increasing or decreasing sympathetic activity. The directing of blood to the muscles during exercise is an important aspect of the stress response, as we shall see later.

'Get set' instructions from the brain via the hormone system

The other means by which the brain instructs the body organs to alter their activity is through the action of hormones released from endocrine glands. Hormones travel in the bloodstream around the body and therefore have access to all the body organs. Each hormone carries a specific message instructing the organs to alter their activity.

Of particular interest to us in considering the stress response are the **adrenal** and **pituitary** glands. The two adrenal glands, one lying on top of each kidney, are the source of several hormones which are released during the stress response (Figure 11). Each gland consists of two parts, an outer part called the **adrenal cortex** and an inner part called the **adrenal medulla**. The medulla produces large quantities of two very similar hormones called **adrenaline** and **noradrenaline**, technically known as catecholamines (pronounced *cat-e-coal-a-means*). The hormone noradrenaline is exactly the same as the neurotransmitter noradrenaline produced by the sympathetic nerve endings. In fact, the adrenal medulla can be regarded as an extension of the sympathetic nervous system. The sympathetic nervous system supplies nerves to the adrenal medulla and controls the release of adrenaline and noradrenaline from it. Although noradrenaline and adrenaline are similar in structure their effects on the body organs are different. This is important in instructing the body organs to prepare for either fighting or fleeing, as we shall see later.

The other part of the adrenal gland, the adrenal cortex, produces different hormones that prepare the body to deal with long-term demands. One of these is **cortisol** which is of particu-

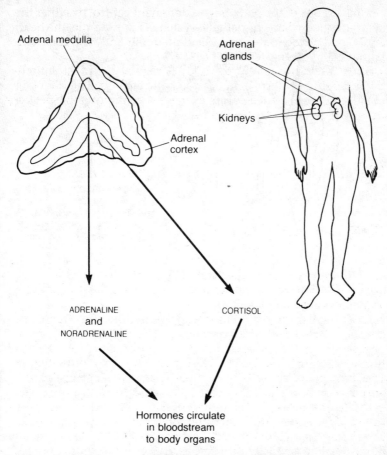

Fig. 11   Adrenal glands; position, structure and hormones produced

lar importance as far as the resistance response is concerned.

The release of most adrenal cortex hormones is controlled by other hormones secreted by the pituitary gland. The pituitary (Figure 12) is known as the 'master endocrine gland' of the body because it controls, by releasing its own hormones, the production and release of hormones from a number of other endocrine glands. The pituitary lies very close to the hypothalamus in the brain and is also under the influence of messages from the hypothalamus. To effect the release of cortisol, for instance, the hypothalamus sends messages to the pituitary which releases

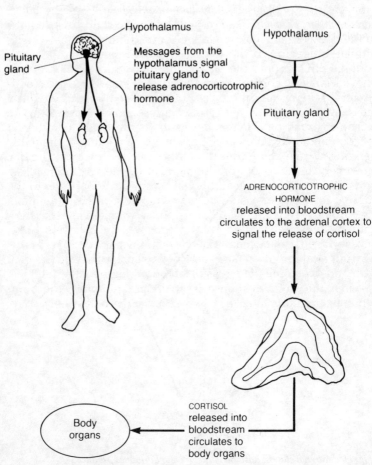

Fig. 12   Mechanism of cortisol release

adrenocorticotrophic hormone (ACTH). This travels in the blood to the adrenal gland and gives the instruction to the adrenal cortex to release cortisol.

Cortisol's main role is to ensure a supply of fuel to active body muscles. It helps to convert stores of fat into energy. Cortisol also makes it easier for the catecholamines to carry out their roles. At normal levels, cortisol aids the body's defence mechanisms to deal with infection or injury.

So the stress response is largely brought about by the action of noradrenaline, adrenaline and cortisol. The brain sends instructions to the body organs mainly via the sympathetic nervous system, ultimately leading to the release of noradrenaline from nerve endings directly onto the organ, and by hormones (noradrenaline, adrenaline, cortisol) from the adrenal glands via the bloodstream to the organ. In the case of noradrenaline this chemical messenger is both a neurotransmitter and a hormone. The reason for such an arrangement is to ensure that the body can react immediately when necessary by using the fast sympathetic nervous system communication line direct to the body organs. However, the effect of noradrenaline at the nerve endings lasts only a few seconds. The additional communication route to the adrenal medulla, releasing both adrenaline and noradrenaline, can prolong and intensify the response initiated by the sympathetic neurotransmitter. This ensures that the body response, once initiated, can be maintained for as long as necessary. In this way physical activity can be sustained to enable the body to deal with and overcome the stressful situation (Figure 13).

When the stress response is no longer required, the brain sends instructions to reduce sympathetic nervous system activ-

Fig. 13   Catecholamine release

ity and to increase parasympathetic nervous system activity. The parasympathetic nervous system then produces acetylcholine which acts on the body organs and this leads to a state of rest and relaxation.

With this array of different neurotransmitters and hormones, it is possible for the brain to initiate the most appropriate organic action by selecting a suitable cocktail of chemical messengers. But how do the body organs know what to do when they are bombarded by different chemical messengers?

How do different chemical messengers bring about different actions?

Noradrenaline and adrenaline both increase heart rate (adrenaline more so than noradrenaline) whilst acetylcholine slows the heart. These different actions take place because the heart, like most other organs of the body, contains different types of receptors, each of which is responsive to only one type of chemical messenger. A receptor is like a locked door which can only be opened by a key (a specific chemical messenger). When a chemical messenger key unlocks its door, chemical processes are triggered that bring about a particular action by the organ.

In the case of the catecholamines, there are two types of receptors called **alpha** (α) and **beta** (β) receptors and both are unlocked by noradrenaline and adrenaline. However, the noradrenaline key unlocks alpha receptors more easily than beta receptors, whilst the opposite is true for adrenaline. So if an organ has a greater number of alpha receptors the action of noradrenaline is dominant, whereas if there are more beta receptors the organ is influenced more by adrenaline. The distribution of alpha and beta receptors in different organs and tissues is shown in the table opposite.

So adrenaline is more effective in increasing heart rate because the heart has more beta than alpha receptors. We can now see why some blood vessels in the body constrict whilst others dilate during sympathetic nervous system activity. If a blood vessel has a predominance of alpha receptors it will respond to noradrenaline and this will lead to constriction. However, if there is a predominance of beta receptors the vessel responds to adrenaline which causes the vessel to dilate. In this way, more

ORGAN/TISSUE	RECEPTORS PRESENT
Heart	more β than α
Most blood vessels	more α than β
Muscle blood vessels	more β than α
Spleen	α
Salivary glands	α
Liver	β
Sugar mobilisation	mostly β
Fat stores	mostly β
Lung airways	β
Noradrenaline more active on **alpha** (α) **Adrenaline** more active on **beta** (β)	

blood can be directed to the right muscles for fight or flight. The airways of the lung have beta receptors which respond to adrenaline, causing the airways to become wider thus allowing air to flow more easily in and out of the lungs.

In the case of the heart there are more beta than alpha receptors present. So whilst both noradrenaline and adrenaline increase heart rate, adrenaline is more effective in doing so because it unlocks the beta receptors more easily. The heart also has receptors responsive to acetylcholine, which lowers the heart rate.

How is the release of the various chemical messengers controlled?

The activity of the autonomic nervous system is controlled by the hypothalamus which receives impulses from many other areas of the brain. One such area, called the **cerebral cortex**, evaluates the information from the senses and decides what response to make; for example, the decision may be, '*I can cope with this situation*'. Another part of the brain called the **limbic system** adds emotion, such as fear or anger, to the response decided by the cortex. The type of emotion evoked depends on how the individual feels about the situation. So the limbic system colours or sets the intensity of the response decided by the cortex, for example, *'I feel angry about this situation'* or *'I am scared of this situation'*.

The final outcome of the interaction of impulses between the cortex and the limbic system is transmitted to the hypothalamus. The hypothalamus translates the decision into a course of action by the body. It organises nerve impulses to the body organs via the sympathetic and parasympathetic nervous systems and hormone release into the blood via the pituitary gland.

'Get set' instructions and coping

As we have explained, activation of the stress response results mainly from the pattern of instructions organised by the hypothalamus and sent via two different systems:

- *Sympathetic nervous system and adrenal medulla (inner part of adrenal gland)*

and

- *Pituitary gland and adrenal cortex (outer part of adrenal gland)*

This is summarised in Figure 14.

We have seen that the expression of the stress response or the way in which we deal with stress has its roots in fight, flight or resistance. We describe below the physical effects of the three responses.

Get set to fight

When the decision is made by the brain to stay and fight, or when a sustained effort is needed to achieve control over a situation, the hypothalamus signals a mainly noradrenaline release via the sympathetic nervous system. It is the predominance of noradrenaline that prepares the body organs for fighting. Aggression, anger and hostility are the emotional hallmarks of fighting behaviour. This may first take the form of a sham attack aimed at frightening off the attacker. In animals such as the cat this may involve baring the teeth, hissing,

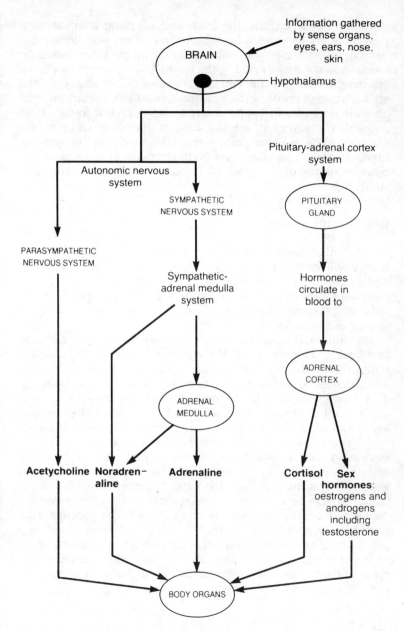

Fig. 14 Biological mechanism of the stress response

showing claws, arching the back and adopting a threatening posture with fur erect. In humans we often see similar behaviours – making threatening noises and gestures, standing erect, showing and clenching the teeth. A sham attack can be an effective defence mechanism in itself since the attacker may call off his aggression or hesitate, think twice before attacking and give the defender the opportunity to strike first. If the attack is for real, the aim is to achieve control and dominance of the situation. The body resources must be mobilised to provide maximal mental alertness and body strength. The stronger and more cunning of the pair of fighters will gain control and survive.

Get set to run away

On the other hand, if there is fear or uncertainty about how things will turn out, or doubts about ability to take control, a decision to run away may be made. The hypothalamus signals a predominantly adrenaline secretion which prepares the body for a fast get-away by increasing heart rate and making plenty of energy available for muscular activity.

Both noradrenaline and adrenaline are needed for fighting and fleeing. However, it is the emotion involved which determines the predominance of either noradrenaline or adrenaline, and thus the action appropriate for either running or fighting. This has given rise to a great deal of confusion over the difference between noradrenaline and adrenaline. Most people say, 'I can feel the adrenaline flowing' when they are stimulated and excited. In fact, it is noradrenaline, not adrenaline, which is associated with arousal and gives rise to feelings of excitement and drive as well as physical strength. For this reason noradrenaline has been named the 'kick' or high performance hormone which in large amounts stimulates special areas in the brain that produce a feeling of pleasure. In contrast, the feelings and sensations associated with high levels of adrenaline are not pleasant. Just think how you felt in the dentist's waiting room or waiting for a surgical operation: that was adrenaline at work, the predominant hormone released for the flight response – you probably felt like running away.

Get set to resist

In situations where demands persist, activity of the pituitary–adrenal cortex system is predominant. Here cortisol is important in keeping up the supply of energy needed by the body for the effort required in the face of long-term demands.

Maintaining the stability of relationships is a long-term demand and this involves the sex hormones oestrogen and the androgens (of which testosterone is the main hormone). Although testosterone is generally known as the male hormone it is also an important sex hormone in women, secreted by the adrenals.

The sex hormones play an important role in our social behaviour; in forming relationships, bonding between the sexes and in mating. It has been shown that sex hormone levels in the body depend on how secure we feel and, for testosterone, how much dominance and control we feel we have in challenging situations. In situations where we feel helpless and a failure, levels of testosterone in the blood fall. This leads to poor motivation to do things and reduced sexual drive in men. High levels are released when we feel elated, secure and loved. This heightens sexual drive and motivates us into action. The role of testosterone in women in these situations is not clear.

GO

Dealing with the demand

When faced with a demand, the sympathetic nervous system initiates the immediate response mainly through the action of noradrenaline. At the same time, it stimulates the adrenal medulla to release its adrenaline and noradrenaline in order to supplement, sustain and prolong the response. These actions are geared mainly to provide energy for muscular activity which increases alertness and strength, and to protect the body from blood loss in the event of injury.

The first objective of the alarm response is to make available adequate oxygen and fuel for conversion into energy to power the muscle action. Extra oxygen needs to be taken from the air by the lungs and then carried by the blood to the exercising muscles. Sugar and fat stores must be mobilised to provide the fuel for energy production.

Getting the right amount of oxygen and fuel to the muscles

The heart beats faster and harder to circulate larger amounts of oxygen and fuel-rich blood to the muscles. The blood vessels supplying the active muscles become wider (dilate) to increase blood flow to its required destination.

In attempting to supply the muscles with the huge amount of oxygen and fuel-rich blood needed for emergency action, the body has a major problem to overcome. There is only a certain amount of blood in the circulation, so if more blood is needed by the muscles then there will be less available for other body organs. Some vital organs, notably the brain, heart muscle and lungs, must always receive a relatively large blood supply and usually this needs to be increased when supporting muscular work. Other organs are less vital in an emergency. The digestive system, kidneys and skin markedly reduce their activity during periods of stress. This means that their blood supply can be reduced, so the blood vessels supplying these areas decrease in diameter and become narrower (constrict). In other words, to supply the body muscles with adequate oxygen and fuels there must be a redistribution of blood throughout the body: take from the non-vital areas and give to the vital.

Obtaining more oxygen

Adrenaline dilates the airways of the lungs so that air will flow more easily in and out of the lungs. Breathing becomes more rapid and deeper so adequate oxygen can be transferred to the blood. The oxygen-carrying capacity of the blood is increased by adding more red blood cells (the oxygen-carrying cells) to the bloodstream. This is done by the sympathetic nervous system stimulation of the spleen which contracts, releasing red blood cells from its store.

Obtaining more fuel

Glucose and fats are quickly mobilised from the body's sugar and fat stores by the action of adrenaline and noradrenaline on the liver and fat tissues. Supplies are maintained by the action of other hormones, including cortisol, released during the stress response.

Increasing alertness and sharpening the senses

Noradrenaline enhances alertness and sensory activity: smell, hearing, taste, touch and sight. The pupils of the eye increase in size to allow more light to enter, thus improving vision, especially in poor light conditions. Hearing becomes more acute and the skin is more sensitive to touch, both clear advantages when fighting. Mental alertness increases, leading amongst other things to quick thinking.

Looking aggressive

An aggressive appearance is achieved by the erection of body hair and tensing of the facial muscles to expose the teeth. This, together with a general tensing of the body and the adoption of an aggressive posture, can give the impression of increased and imposing size aimed at frightening the opponent into retreat. Noradrenaline is involved with these responses.

Reducing activity of non-vital functions

Whilst fighting and fleeing, non-vital functions such as digestion and urine formation which are not required slow down or stop.

Actions of Adrenaline and Noradrenaline

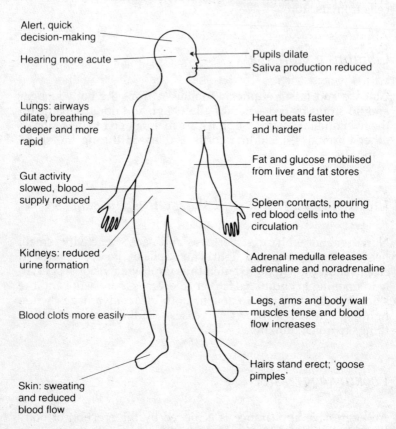

Alert, quick decision-making

Hearing more acute

Lungs: airways dilate, breathing deeper and more rapid

Gut activity slowed, blood supply reduced

Kidneys: reduced urine formation

Blood clots more easily

Skin: sweating and reduced blood flow

Pupils dilate

Saliva production reduced

Heart beats faster and harder

Fat and glucose mobilised from liver and fat stores

Spleen contracts, pouring red blood cells into the circulation

Adrenal medulla releases adrenaline and noradrenaline

Legs, arms and body wall muscles tense and blood flow increases

Hairs stand erect; 'goose pimples'

Fig. 15   Effect of sympathetic-adrenal medulla system activation

Tensing the muscles

The catecholamines increase the tenseness of the body muscles, keeping them partially contracted ready to spring into action. The strength of contraction of the muscles is also increased, particularly by noradrenaline.

Minimising blood loss due to injury

Another set of alarm responses is aimed at reducing loss of blood in case of injury during the attack or escape. Noradrenaline increases the speed at which the blood clots. This, together with the constriction of the skin blood vessels in the blood redistribution process, means that there is less chance of serious blood loss if wounded.

Mending wounds

Cortisol is released during and after the alarm reaction to reduce inflammation and assist wound healing so that injured tissues can be mended as soon as possible.

Suppression of the allergic reaction

Cortisol suppresses the body's allergic reaction. This is beneficial when fighting or fleeing since dust and other irritants can cause breathlessness, runny nose and eyes and, as a consequence, reduced performance.

Both the alarm response and resistance response operate together to assist the body in defending itself. In persistent, distressful situations we might feel like running away but cannot. Instead we must stay and cope as best we can. This can lead to lengthy periods of cortisol release. On the other hand, when faced with a non life-threatening demand that will not go away, we might feel like fighting. However, the nature of the situation may not allow it, so we bottle up our feelings of irritation and anger. This can lead to an overproduction of noradrenaline. Our feelings or emotions can and do affect the activation of the stress response. This is examined next.

Your emotions are revealed in your blood chemistry

To illustrate how our emotions are related to the levels of

Actions of Cortisol

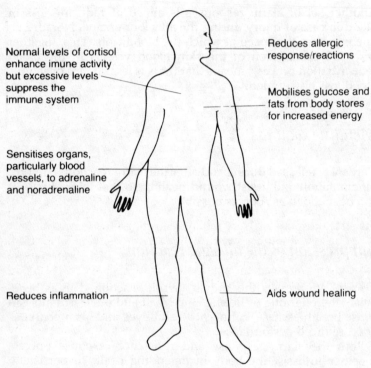

Fig. 16   Effect of sympathetic-adrenal cortex system activation

noradrenaline, adrenaline and cortisol, let us take two situations. A man flying from Heathrow to New York had a blood sample taken just before the flight. The sample was tested for noradrenaline and adrenaline levels. At New York he hired a car to drive downtown. Another blood sample was taken before he drove off and was again tested for noradrenaline and adrenaline levels.

From these results the levels of noradrenaline and adrenaline can be related to the way the man was feeling at the time. Where he was not in control of the situation – a passenger on the plane – his emotions produced the relative levels of adrenaline (high) and noradrenaline (low). Having reached his destination and probably relieved to be on the ground, he got into his car, drove

	LEVELS IN BLOOD: NA A	SITUATION AND EMOTION
Before flight	Low High	Not in control of aeroplane – uncertainty about outcome of flight
Before driving	High Low	In control of driving the car but must make decisions to drive safely in a potentially hostile environment

NA = Noradrenaline   A = Adrenaline

off and felt in control of the driving situation. Once again, his emotions were reflected in the levels of noradrenaline (high) and adrenaline (low). So the level of chemicals associated with the stress response is very much determined by our emotions.

Let us take another example. Blood samples were taken from two experienced motor rally drivers before each attempted a rally circuit and again when they had finished. The blood samples were analysed for levels of noradrenaline, adrenaline and cortisol. Below are the results of the blood analysis of the winner and loser driver. The levels of hormones shown are those after the rally, compared with those before the start of the competition.

Can you pick the winner by looking at these blood analysis results?

Driver	Noradrenaline	Adrenaline	Cortisol
A	Small increase	Large increase	Large increase
B	Large increase	Small increase	No change

Rally driving is not a race against other competitors but against time. At the end of the race, each driver will have judged how well he had performed and whether he felt he had mastered the course. The winner's blood chemistry should indicate that he felt he had mastered the circuit and performed well, so his noradrenaline levels should be higher than those of the loser. Also the winner's adrenaline and cortisol levels should be lower than those of the loser, who most likely felt he had not mastered the circuit and therefore did not expect to win. So looking at the results, driver B would be the winner. In fact he was. It is interesting to learn that the noradrenaline levels were higher at the end of the race for both drivers, reflecting the increased alertness and physical effort required for the race.

The chemical messenger league table below and Figure 17 summarise the relationship between how we feel and the release of the stress response hormones.

Chemical messenger league table

APPRAISAL OF SITUATION	DOMINANT PART OF STRESS RESPONSE	CHEMICAL MESSENGER(S) ORDER OF DOMINANCE
'I can cope' 'I am in control' 'I have mastered this'	Alarm 'Fight' aspect	1 **Noradrenaline** 2 Adrenaline
'This is too demanding' 'Can I cope?' 'I fear failure'	Alarm 'Flight' aspect leading to resistance	1 **Adrenaline** 2 *Cortisol* 3 Noradrenaline
'I feel helpless' 'I am not in control' 'I have failed'	Resistance	1 **Cortisol** 2 Adrenaline

Power of the alarm response

The stress response allows us to produce extremes of human performance; speed, strength and stamina. There are numerous stories describing tremendous feats of power during activation of the alarm reaction. A woman achieved the strength to lift a car, releasing her trapped child. A man racing for cover during an air

EMOTIONS/ BHEAVIOURS	CHEMICAL MESSENGERS/ HORMONES	AMOUNT AND DIRECTION OF CHANGE FROM 'NORMAL' LEVELS
ANGER AGGRESSION 'FIGHT'	NORADRENALINE ADRENALINE TESTOSTERONE CORTISOL	large increase small increase small increase little or no change
FEAR WITHDRAWL 'FLIGHT'	ADRENALINE CORTISOL NORADRENALINE TESTOSTERONE	large increase increase small increase little or no change
DEPRESSION LOSS OF CONTROL SUBMISSION	CORTISOL ADRENALINE NORADRENALINE TESTOSTERONE	large increase little or no change little or no change decrease
SERENITY RELAXATION MEDITATION	NORADRENALINE ADRENALINE CORTISOL TESTOSTERONE	decrease decrease little or no change little or no change
ELATION SECURITY LOVE AND SUPPORT	TESTOSTERONE NORADRENALINE ADRENALINE CORTISOL	increase decrease decrease decrease

Fig. 17   Relationship between how you feel and some of the hormones released in your body

raid did not realise that he scaled a ten foot wall in his dash for
safety. If there had not been an emergency, neither the man nor
woman would have had the physical strength to perform these
feats.

Athletes and sportsmen use the fight response to 'psych'
themselves up before races and events. Observe Olympic
weightlifters. Notice how they pace up and down preparing to
attack the weight as though it were a sabre-toothed tiger that
they are about to take on in battle. Look at the aggression and
hostility in their faces and behaviour. Ready for action, they
grasp the bar, 'attack', and lift.

Athletes often drive themselves to the limits of human performance. To achieve this, they must reduce the pain that arises
during intense muscle activity. When they continue to perform
even though they should really stop, a group of chemicals called
endorphins are released in the brain to suppress the pain
associated with the body's efforts. Joggers and long distance
runners owe their sustained activity to endorphins which produce a euphoric feeling. This may be one reason why joggers
say they feel so good after a run when in fact they often look
terrible! Being able to pass through the pain barrier is essential
for survival if we are in a life or death situation and need to
continue our effort until we are safe.

4 Signs of Stress

Recognising the signs of activity of your stress response and identifying the position of your stress balance are essential if you are to reduce distress, avoid ugly stress and make stress work for you. Your knowledge of the biology of the stress response can now be put to the test.

Linking the physiology of the stress response to the signs of stress

Most signs of stress can be explained by looking at the physiological actions of the stress response in the body. For example, a sign of stress is cold hands and feet. Why? The skin temperature of the hands and feet is determined by the amount of blood flowing into these areas, and when the flow is significantly reduced, the hands and feet will feel cold. There are a number of factors that can change skin blood flow, such as environmental temperature, but one action that certainly does is the stress response. If you remember, there is a redistribution of blood flow in the body during the alarm response, taking blood away from non-essential areas and diverting it to the muscles and other essential regions. The skin is a non-essential area so the sympathetic nervous system sends messages to the blood vessels of the skin instructing them to constrict. This leads to reduced blood flow and therefore reduced heat, which results in cold hands and feet. Using this as an example, it is possible to explain how and why the signs of stress arise. By referring to the actions of adrenaline, noradrenaline and cortisol, described in the previous chapter, we show the effects on the body of stress response activation when the stress balance is in the normal zone and no stress is experienced. It then becomes possible to explain what happens to the body when the stress response is

overactivated and the stress balance tips out of the normal zone, giving rise to distress or eustress. This is the topic of the next chapter.

A letter of distress

The following are extracts from a letter we received from a man after he read a news article featuring our work;

'For almost thirty years I was employed as a Sales Manager for a local manufacturing company and during the last three years of my employment was promoted to Sales Director at a critical time in the company's history. At this time we were faced with 'cheap' (not necessarily inferior quality) imported products and in consequence the company could not compete and faced what became a slow but inevitable decline from 400 workers to 36.

I was taking sole responsibility for sales. You can probably appreciate the attendant anxiety and frustration I personally experienced. Many were the long nights when *I couldn't sleep, lying there worrying* about how I could maintain sales, to arrest the decline of the company. *Frequently sweating with anxiety* and *constantly aware of a heavy throbbing heart-beat in my ear* when my head rested on the pillow. Severe *angina* forced me to retire early.

Nowadays I find I am easily under stress even when doing simple tasks. *I have had to break off when writing this letter as I can feel tensions building up in me.*

I have not worked for 4½ years and *see no prospects of becoming employable again.* Please keep pointing out to the general public the dangers of stress situations as I feel sure that some individuals will heed your valuable advice and hopefully will then not have to *suffer "the indignity"* of being unemployable for the rest of their lives, as I have done.'

The sections shown in italics describe some of the signs of bad and ugly distress, both physical and mental.

Signs of distress

PHYSICAL

Aware of heart beating, palpitations

Breathlessness, lump in the throat, rapid shallow breathing

Dry mouth, 'butterflies' in stomach, indigestion, nausea

Diarrhoea, constipation, flatulence

General muscle tenseness particularly of the jaws, grinding of teeth

Clenched fists, hunched shoulders, general muscle aches and pains, cramps

Restless, hyperactive, nail biting, finger drumming, foot tapping, hands shaking

Tired, fatigued, lethargic, exhausted, sleep difficulties, feeling faint, headaches, frequent illnesses such as colds

Sweaty especially palms and upper lip, hot flushed feeling

Cold hands and feet

Frequent desire to urinate

Overeating, loss of appetite, increased cigarette smoking

Increased alcohol consumption, loss of interest in sex

MENTAL

Distressed, worried, upset, tearful, deflated, feelings of helplessness and hopelessness, hysterical, withdrawn, feeling unable to cope, anxious, depressed

Impatient, easily irritated and aggravated, angry, hostile, aggressive

Frustrated, bored, inadequate, guilty, rejected, neglected, insecure, vulnerable

Loss of interest in self-appearance, health, diet, sex; low self-esteem, and loss of interest in others

Polyphasic (doing too many things at once), rushed

Failing to finish tasks before moving on to the next

Difficulty in thinking clearly, concentrating and making decisions, forgetful, lack of creativity, irrational; procrastinating, difficulty in starting to do things

Prone to making silly mistakes and having accidents

Having so much to do and not knowing where to start so ending up doing nothing or going from task to task and not completing anything

Hypercritical, inflexible, unreasonable, over-reactive non-productive, poor efficiency

NB: This list is not exhaustive and some of the mental signs could be regarded as physical signs and vice versa.

Signs of eustress

Clearly, an absence of the signs and symptoms of distress indicates that you are not suffering the bad effects of stress. The signs of eustress paint a picture of how you might feel when you are harnessing the positive aspects of the stress response. You might feel and appear:

Euphoric, stimulated, thrilled, excited

Helpful, understanding, sociable, friendly, loving, happy

Calm, controlled, confident

Creative, effective, efficient

Clear and rational in thought, decisive

Industrious, lively, productive, jolly, often smiling

Looking at the lists and thinking about your own experience, it is striking how many different signs there are. This is because the stress response involves so many body organs and activities. As was pointed out earlier, the stress reaction is a general response by the body to any demand made upon it. However, some body systems are more involved than others, for example, the heart and circulation, the lungs and the muscles. So when we ask the participants at our workshops to construct a list of their signs of physical stress, such things as awareness of heart beating, racing heart, heart palpitations (irregular beating), heart pounding against chest, fast, shallow and irregular breathing and tense muscles are virtually in every column under 'distress'. So too are other signs such as sweaty palms, butterflies in the stomach and a desire to urinate. Less commonly, we see items that describe general muscle tenseness such as jaws clenched tightly together, grinding of teeth, clenched fists and hunched shoulders, cold hands and feet. We believe there are two reasons for this. Firstly, most people do not usually associate these signs with distress and secondly, many people are under distress so much of the time that these activities have become habitual and are therefore never associated with distress. This raises an important point. *We must all learn to listen to our body and to read and take notice of the messages it is sending.*

Similarly for the mental signs of distress, there are many items that would appear on most lists such as feeling impatient, rushed, irritable, frustrated, bored, neglected, helpless, tearful, worried, loss of appetite, overeating, loss of interest in sex, inability to concentrate and trying to do too many things at once. Others such as reduced ability to be creative, difficulty in making decisions and proneness to silly mistakes and accidents are less frequently listed. Interestingly, the mental signs list is nearly always longer than that for the physical signs. We are more aware of how we feel emotionally than of the physical signs that accompany these emotions. This emphasises the need for us to take more notice of our body and to realise that what happens in the mind can affect the body.

Another interesting observation we have made is that when we ask participants to construct a list of the mental and physical signs of stress, their lists are made up almost entirely of signs of distress with virtually none for eustress. This illustrates the fact that most people simply think of stress as bad and do not usually associate creativity, efficiency, effectiveness, mental alertness and so on with the stress response. They never think of stress as being good as well as bad. No one would argue with the fact that stress is good when it saves our life and defends us from real harm. However, since such situations are few and far between we tend not to recognise them nor use the benefits that the stress response can provide.

The outward signs of hormone activity

We have described how the stress response is mediated via different chemicals, notably noradrenaline, adrenaline and cortisol, so that different body actions can take place. It is possible to identify those signs in the body and mind which are produced by the action of noradrenaline, adrenaline or cortisol.

Noradrenaline

Noradrenaline is associated with aggression and fighting behaviour as shown by changes in facial muscle tenseness and drawing back of the lips to show the teeth which are clenched together. The back and shoulder muscles tense (hunched shoulders) and the fists clench. Hairs stand more erect; this is seen as 'goose pimples' since humans have relatively little body hair compared to other animals. All this action is to make us look more threatening and hostile. Also, the skin blood vessels constrict, and the palms of the hands, the feet and the upper lip become sweaty. The pupil of the eye dilates, mental alertness increases, thinking and decision-making become quicker and performance improves. Noradrenaline produces a feeling of pleasantness and excitement in the absence of irritation, anger and hostility.

Adrenaline

Adrenaline on the other hand is more orientated toward preparing the body for a quick getaway. Heart action increases and can be felt as a pounding in the chest. This is sometimes erratic and described as heart palpitations. Blood supply to the vital organs and skeletal muscles increases so it is necessary for noradrenaline to reduce the supply to the non-vital organs such as the gut and skin. This, together with a reduction in activity of the gut, gives the feeling of butterflies and knots in the tummy. A 'cold sweat' is experienced when sweat is secreted onto the surface of a cold skin. Feelings of uncertainty, worry, insecurity and anxiety are examples of the results of adrenaline activity.

Cortisol

Outward physical signs that cortisol is at work are difficult to see although frequent colds, allergies or asthma could be indicators. However, the mental signs are clear enough; feelings of failure, helplessness, hopelessness, chronic anxiety, depression.

Recognising stress in others as well as yourself

The main purpose of this book is to help you learn to recognise and manage stress in yourself. But it is also important that you can identify the signs of stress in others; your family, friends and work colleagues.

Being alert to the signs of distress in others will help you to reduce relationship problems and maintain a creative and productive office and organisation. At work it would be foolish to pile more tasks onto your colleague who is rushing around trying to do too many things at once and becoming impatient, easily irritated at trivial things and snappy with workmates. Or to ignore an overloaded colleague who has problems at home and perhaps withdraws, becomes uncharacteristically quiet and looks depressed. Watch out also for the colleague who becomes frustrated and bored because there is too little to do and who feels her abilities and talents are not being adequately used.

Not all the signs are exclusively signs of stress

Care must be taken in interpreting the signs of stress since many can be due to other factors. For instance, cold hands can be due to winter weather! A low external temperature is a physical stressor because it activates the body's stress response, within the normal zone, so that a normal body temperature can be maintained. Unless the temperatures are extreme and potentially life-threatening, most people would not say they felt 'stressed' because of them. So a person might have cold hands but not feel emotionally stressed at the time. Furthermore, some diseases of the circulation can lead to poor blood flow into the hands, resulting in coldness.

Signs such as back and neck pain, headaches, muscular aches and pains, spasms and cramps, constipation, diarrhoea, indigestion and nausea can all arise for reasons other than stress. It is when we find a number of these signs occurring together that we can often attribute them to stress.

Hidden signs

It is impossible for us to see blood glucose and fat levels changing, more red cells pouring into the bloodstream, blood clotting more easily or wound healing processes being stimulated when the stress response is at work. These signs are hidden from our eyes but not from the scientist who, with an array of highly sophisticated instruments, can spot and measure the internal actions of the stress response.

Unfortunately many of the hidden signs outwardly rear their ugly heads only when it is too late. Their continued or frequent action can lead to ill health and death and only then can they be seen! The purpose of being *Stresswise* is to take heed of outward physical and mental signs of stress and to *take preventive action before it is too late!*

5 Stress and Health

The stress response involves all body functions so too much distress overtaxing our adaptive resources can lead to exhaustion, a variety of health problems and can even be fatal. It has been estimated that at least 75% of illness reported to GPs is stress related. Some doctors have even suggested that almost all illness and premature deaths can be associated with distress. This is not hard to believe when you consider that stress affects all our body systems including our defence and immune mechanisms. We are also more prone to accidents when we are distressed.

Industry and commerce have seen how distress can affect productivity and profits. Surveys and studies have estimated that 100 million working days are lost each year due to distress-related illness and absenteeism, costing the country around £3 billion per annum. Companies pay the price of distress by loss of personnel through resignation or premature retirement. Apart from the personal effects of distress-related ill health, there are also the demands it places on the family. Disability, medical treatment and sick leave from work pose varied and incalculable demands on the family's and nation's caring resources.

Many researchers and doctors now believe that excessive, frequent and prolonged action of the stress response, particularly without the normal outlet for the accompanying physical activity, can lead to a variety of disorders and diseases. This is most clearly seen in the cardiovascular system which is heavily involved in the alarm reaction. The digestive system is also very vulnerable. Recent research has shown how cortisol can adversely affect the immune system. Chronic stimulation of this system by cortisol reduces the body's ability to deal with infection and increases susceptibility to diseases such as cancer.

The effects mentioned so far are physical but the emotional diseases, such as anxiety and depression, are perhaps the more obvious consequences of distress. Furthermore our behaviour and lifestyle frequently change when we are distressed. Altered eating, smoking and drinking patterns and drug abuse bring their own problems and add to the health risks normally associated with these behaviours. Some distress-related disorders and diseases are shown in the table below. These range from symptoms that are simply unpleasant and uncomfortable to more serious illnesses that can be disabling, life-threatening and fatal.

Some distress-related disorders and diseases

CARDIOVASCULAR SYSTEM

Coronary heart disease (angina and heart attacks)
Hypertension (high blood pressure)
Strokes
Migraine

DIGESTIVE SYSTEM

Indigestion
Nausea
Heartburn
Stomach and duodenal ulcers
Ulcerative colitis
Irritable bowel syndrome
Diarrhoea
Constipation
Flatulence

MUSCLES AND JOINTS

Headaches
Cramps
Muscle spasm
Back pain
Neck pain

OTHERS

Diabetes
Cancers
Rheumatoid arthritis
Allergies
Asthma
Common cold and flu

Sexual disorders – reduced sex drive, premature ejaculation,
                       failure to reach orgasm, infertility
Skin disorders
Sleep disorders

BEHAVIOURAL

Overeating – obesity
Loss of appetite – anorexia
Increased cigarette smoking
Increased caffeine intake
Increased alcohol consumption
Drug abuse

EMOTIONAL

Anxiety, including fears, phobias and obsessions.
Depression

Why is it that a response evolved to save life and improve performance ends up actually making us less efficient and becomes a potential killer? To answer this we must go back to many of the points made earlier in Chapter 3. In brief, the stress response was evolved primarily to preserve our lives in the face of life-threatening situations in a physically hostile environment. It was ideal for the threats and challenges faced by our early ancestors, but today we rarely face physical dangers such as an attack by a wild animal. Rather, we live in a society involving complex social interactions. The threats we perceive are to our self-esteem, and the security of our relationships and jobs.

We know *homo sapiens* has existed for around forty thousand years in essentially the same biological form as we are today. The urbanised, industrialised, high technology era is a very recent phenomenon in this evolutionary period but has presented the greatest amount of environmental change in a relatively short time. We still have the same biological mechanism – the stress response – to deal with a very different environment. No wonder we suffer the consequences of an outdated biological system which is largely inappropriate for today's demands and pressures.

Today we are bombarded with a continuous stream of emotional threats and challenges and if our beliefs lead us regularly to perceive these as stressors, *real or imaginary*, then we face the consequences of ill health and death as a result of over-using our stress response.

How the stress response can lead to ill health and death

The stress response, angina and heart attacks

Excessive levels of noradrenaline can lead to heart and circulatory diseases, as noradrenaline's most potent action is to constrict blood vessels. During the alarm reaction, this increases the blood pressure, so the heart must work harder to overcome the higher pressure in order to circulate the blood. At the same time, noradrenaline steps up the heart rate, further increasing the heart's workload. A higher workload requires more oxygen and glucose and this is delivered to the heart muscle (known as the myocardium) via the coronary arteries. However, in those people with coronary artery disease* this could be a problem.

In coronary artery disease one or more of the coronary arteries becomes partially obstructed by the build-up of a substance known as **plaque**. This furring up is known as atherosclerosis and can lead to myocardial ischaemia (myocardium poorly supplied with blood) (Figure 18). If a coronary artery becomes severely narrowed, sufficient blood cannot reach the heart muscle to support its workload. The resultant myocardial ischaemia produces a pain across the chest known as angina pectoris. This usually arises during physical exertion or emo-

---

* It is thought that most people in western societies have some degree of coronary artery disease. For the majority this will never cause problems but others suffer angina or have a heart attack. Unfortunately it is not easy to predict who is at risk without performing special medical tests. These tests are expensive and carry an element of risk so unless there are particular medical reasons for doing so, 'healthy' individuals would not be referred for this investigation. If you have chest pains or are in doubt you should see your doctor.

Coronary arteries deliver blood to heart muscle

When heart workload increases more oxygen and fuels/glucose are required by the muscle but because of the plaque not enough blood can get through to the muscle to satisfy its needs so this area of muscle becomes ischaemic

HEART

Cross section of artery

Plaque

blood

Plaque

Only area through which blood can flow

Coronary artery

Fig. 18   Coronary artery disease

tional stress and is relieved by resting or reducing stress. Those people who suffer from angina might consider themselves 'lucky'. They have been given a warning sign that their coronary arteries are becoming progressively and dangerously narrowed. With the right medication and change in lifestyle their disease can be managed successfully.

For many, however, the first sign of their coronary artery disease is an unexpected heart attack. Here there is a sudden and severe reduction in the blood supply to the myocardium and part of it dies. If only a small amount of heart muscle is affected the victim usually survives and the dead part of the heart turns into a scar. This is usually the case for about half of those who have a heart attack. Their myocardial damage is not extensive enough for complications to arise and serious problems may never occur in future as long as attention is paid to living a healthy and careful lifestyle. However, for the other half their heart attack is fatal. In many of these cases a coronary artery is suddenly blocked, leading to cessation of blood supply to the myocardium. This can cause the death of a large part of the heart muscle. Furthermore, the oxygen-starved myocardium can send the heart into ventricular fibrillation (chaotic rapid contractions of the main pumping chambers of the heart) rendering the heart useless as a pump. Under these circumstances, the circulation stops and the victim dies unless the fibrillation is quickly corrected by using a cardiac defibrillator. This device stops the heart beating, thus allowing the heart's natural pacemaker to take control again.

So excessive levels of noradrenaline released during anger and rage could raise the heart's workload to a point where myocardial ischaemia could be fatal. Those people who have angina or have suffered a heart attack are particularly vulnerable.

Noradrenaline can affect its victims in a number of other ways. Some researchers believe that excessive noradrenaline can cause rupture of the plaque, leading to a sudden blockage of the coronary artery. It is thought this occurs because noradrenaline may constrict the small blood vessels that grow into the plaque to provide it with nourishment. Over time, this can lead to plaque necrosis (death of the cells) and eventually plaque rupture. The exposed material of the plaque presents a surface on which a blood clot can form (Figure 19). Clot formation is also encouraged by noradrenaline (remember an action of noradrenaline is to help prevent blood loss if cut during a fight!). The blood supply to the myocardium is suddenly cut off resulting in a heart attack.

Angina and heart attacks can also occur in the absence of significant coronary artery disease. High levels of noradrenaline can cause muscular spasm of the coronary arteries which close up, thereby reducing or stopping blood flow to the myocardium.

Excessive levels of noradrenaline and adrenaline are also known to damage the heart muscle cells directly, reducing the contractile ability of the heart. Post-mortem examination of the

1 Blood vessels grow into plaque to provide nourishment

Plaque

2 Noradrenaline constricts blood vessels so plaque is inadequately nourished. After a time the cells of the plaque die (necrosis)

3 Plaque cap ruptures at edges. Blood clot forms which almost or entirely blocks the artery. Noradrenaline increases ease of clotting

Fig. 19   Plaque rupture and clot formation

hearts of patients who have died from a tumour of the adrenal medulla reveals extensive heart muscle damage. This is caused by the extremely high levels of noradrenaline and adrenaline produced by the tumour. Furthermore, excessive catecholamine levels can directly trigger abnormal electrical activity in the heart, resulting in abnormal rhythms which may cause fatal ventricular fibrillation.

Stress and silent heart attacks

The recent development of sophisticated heart monitoring in-struments has made it possible to record every heartbeat during a 24-hour period while a person goes about his normal activities. The recordings of the heartbeats, known as the electrocardio-gram or ECG for short, are picked up by wires stuck to the chest and recorded on a cassette in a special recorder worn around the waist. The tape is played back through an analyser that detects abnormal rhythms and possible myocardial ischaemia.

We made a 24-hour recording of the heartbeat of a woman

taking part in an experiment to investigate factors affecting heart activity. At 8.30pm there was a change in the shape of part of the ECG, known as the ST segment. Changes in this segment usually indicate myocardial ischaemia. The woman had been asked to keep a 24-hour diary of activities and feelings during the experiment and at around 8.30pm she had recorded a short period of intense emotional arousal soon after she missed her last train home. She reported, 'I was very angry with myself for getting the departure time wrong. I thought it was 8.30, in fact it was 8.15.' The woman had no diagnosed heart disease nor any indication of heart problems yet at 8.30pm a minor myocardial ischaemic episode occurred. What is more, she was completely unaware of it happening and for this reason such an attack is known as silent myocardial ischaemia.

Many experiments have used this technique to assess the effect of stress on the heart function of normal healthy individuals and it appears that stress can cause abnormal heart rhythms and myocardial ischaemia severe enough to induce a small silent heart attack!

Stress, cholesterol and heart disease

Noradrenaline, adrenaline, cortisol and other hormones help mobilise glucose and fats from the body stores, so increasing blood glucose, cholesterol and triglyceride (fat) levels. A high level of circulating blood cholesterol is considered a coronary heart disease risk factor because cholesterol is a major component of plaque. Damage to the inner lining of the blood vessel increases susceptibility to the plaque-forming process by allowing cholesterol to penetrate into the blood vessel wall. There is some evidence to suggest that high circulating levels of noradrenaline and adrenaline can cause this damage.

It is popularly believed that cholesterol from food is solely responsible for elevating blood cholesterol levels but it is not always realised that far more is produced during periods of stress than can be obtained from the diet.

A number of research studies have shown how blood cholesterol levels rise during periods of stress. In one such experiment blood cholesterol was measured in two groups of accountants throughout a period of about six months. During this time the accountants were asked to keep a record of their lifestyle (diet, exercise and so on) and also how much pressure and stress they experienced. Accountants were chosen for the experiment because they have to work to deadlines. In fact, one group were tax accountants and had one deadline to meet in April whilst the others were corporate accountants who had deadlines to meet in January and April. Figure 20 shows that, for both groups, there is a peak in blood cholesterol levels coinciding with the deadlines; one for the tax accountants and two for the corporate accountants. Almost all the accountants reported feeling distressed around the time of the deadlines but there was no significant change in diet or exercise reported.

GROUP 1: 18 tax accountants with work deadline in April

GROUP 2: 22 corporate accountants with additional deadline in January

Adapted from:
Friedman & Rosenman Circ. 17.852–861 1958

Fig. 20   Average blood cholesterol levels in accountants as they face deadlines

When the level of fat in the blood increases, the blood becomes thicker and more viscous. This also occurs when more red cells are pumped into the circulation from the spleen during the stress response. The heart must work harder to circulate thicker blood, therefore myocardial oxygen consumption increases. Another problem with thicker blood is that red blood cells can form a 'sludge' which may block small blood vessels. Sludging in the very small blood vessels of the heart and brain can lead to a heart attack or stroke respectively.

Thus a good case can be made for the involvement of the stress response in circulatory diseases: coronary heart disease, sudden cardiac death, hypertension and strokes. These diseases may result from the interaction between stress and other factors such as diet, smoking and Type A behaviour.

Stress response and the immune system

Perhaps one of the most significant effects of prolonged stress is the suppression of the immune system brought about by cortisol. In excess amounts, cortisol is known to decrease the number of circulating lymphocytes and eosinophils (blood cells which help fight infection), cause the thymus and lymph nodes (areas where the lymphocytes are manufactured) to shrivel up, and depress the production of antibodies (agents which fight infection). Thus the immune system is weakened and the ability to fight infection is reduced, so common colds and influenza may be experienced more frequently. In addition, the body becomes more susceptible to immune system-related diseases such as rheumatoid arthritis, allergies, asthma and cancers.

Stress response and other disorders and diseases

Eating whilst the digestive system is partially shut down during stress can lead to a number of problems such as indigestion, nausea and diarrhoea. In addition, many of the body's healing processes are affected. For example, damage to the stomach lining is normally quickly rectified. However, chronic distress slows down the healing processes which leads to prolonged erosion of the wall by acid, resulting in the formation of an ulcer.

The situation is further aggravated because more acid is produced by the stomach during the stress response.

Excessive chronic stress can also lead to weight loss, insomnia, hyperactivity (shakiness and jumpiness) and sexual disorders. Anxiety and fear are often associated with sexual problems; impotence and premature ejaculation in men and difficulty in reaching orgasm in women. Worrying about events, such as job interviews and examinations, can lead to menstrual cycle irregularities, loss of interest in sexual activities and reduced fertility. Emotional factors are thought to account for around 25% of all infertility problems.

Persistently high blood sugar levels can occur during prolonged distress, leading to diabetes. The depletion of endorphins (pain suppressors) during chronic stress makes pain more apparent in diseases such as arthritis. Back and neck pain, headaches and migraines, brought on by prolonged muscle tension during the stress response are less bearable. Chronic distress can also lead to severe anxiety and depression, disabling mental illnesses, nervous breakdown and suicide.

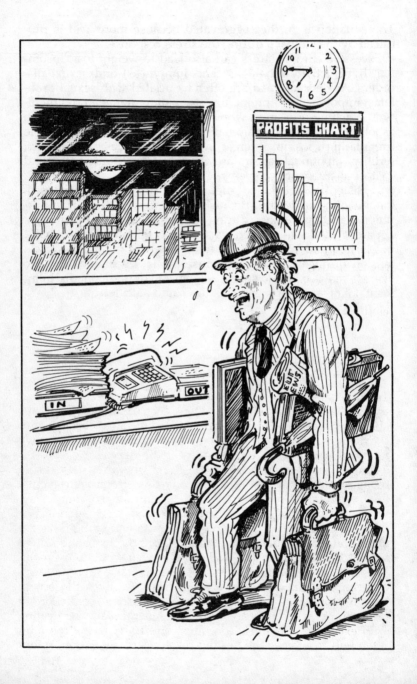

6 Stress and Performance

Life would be dull and uninteresting if we did not experience the stimulating feeling of eustress associated with the challenge of physical performance and the testing of our skills and mental ability. In this case, the effects of a challenge will not usually lead to ill health, provided the energy generated by the stress response is used appropriately and we feel in control and able to cope. However, too few demands or excessive demands (either one major or several minor demands) can overtax our ability to cope effectively, even in those who have good coping ability. This is particularly so if these demands occur frequently or are prolonged. The effect of stress on performance is illustrated in Figure 21.

The performance curve

Too little stimulation, too few demands and challenges can lead to boredom, frustration and a feeling that we are not using our abilities to the full. This situation will tip the stress balance into the distress zone and result in poor performance in whatever we do. Similarly, excessive demands can be very distressful, for example, work overload, extreme time pressure, inescapable demands imposed by others, and too many stressful life events. Such demands can make us feel that control is slipping away, we start doubting our ability to cope and consequently our performance suffers. This is particularly so where the tasks are complicated, unusual or unfamiliar. On the other hand where we perceive demands and challenges as well within our capabilities and we feel confident in handling the task, then performance improves and reaches a peak. However, even those who usually cope well will inevitably suffer some reduction of performance when they are under extreme pressure and dealing with excessive demands. Too much effort and trying too hard often fails to achieve the desired result. Working flat out under

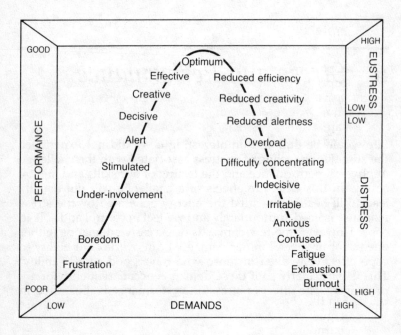

Fig. 21   Stress and performance

high pressure (that is, many demands) to get things done is not always the right strategy, as can be seen in Figure 21. This way of working may achieve goals in the short term but working at high pressure over a long period will inevitably take its toll on the performance, productivity, relationships and health of most people.

Working in this way is like running a car without stopping to service it. As long as the tank is filled with petrol the engine will keep running but what happens when the tyres lose air and the spark plugs are not changed? Performance drops. Eventually, if the car continues to be driven without any attention, it will break down.

Some people can successfully concentrate a high workload into a short period and achieve effective results but they know when to stop for a break. They take the necessary time to relax and recharge their batteries.

Peak performance

Maximum performance is achieved on the top part of the upward slope of the performance curve where we feel stimulated, alert, are better at making decisions, are more creative and effective in achieving results. Peak performance is reached when we are dealing with just the right number and types of demands and challenges and we feel confident and well able to handle them.

On the slippery slope to disaster

However, if demands and pressures continue to increase beyond this point, our coping resources become steadily over-taxed and our performance starts to decline. We hit the downward slope of the curve. If this continues then we could find ourselves on the slippery slope of the distress zone; destination anxiety, fatigue, exhaustion and mental breakdown, often referred to as 'burnout'.

Noradrenaline and adrenaline again

Looking back at the actions of the stress response and the effects of noradrenaline and adrenaline, it is clear to see how stress affects performance. Noradrenaline increases alertness, improves concentration, mental ability, learning and decision-making and it makes us feel good. Adrenaline has none of these benefits and makes us feel awful. It can make us forget things more easily, reduce concentration and decision-making ability.

Working in the eustress zone means having a predominance of noradrenaline activity. But do not be alarmed after reading the chapter on how noradrenaline can lead to ill health and death! Working in the eustress zone means activating the stress response by just the right amount so that you feel confident in dealing with your demands and challenges. The amount of noradrenaline released in the body to achieve this is not harmful; it is only when excessive amounts of noradrenaline are released that harm arises. Of course, being on the eustress side of the normal stress zone means keeping away from the distress zone as much as possible. This can be done by reducing or limiting demands and building up coping resources.

Stress and the performance of industry, commerce and the professions

The costs of distress in terms of health, performance and productivity are all too clear for the individual but the cost to organisations, industry, commerce and the professions is often not appreciated. Considerable financial losses can result from absenteeism due to stress-related disorders and loss of trained personnel through early retirement or premature death. But these calculable costs represent only the tip of a huge financial iceberg. What is difficult to estimate is the cost of distress hidden under the waterline (Figure 22).

Furthermore individuals in the distress zone are more accident-prone. Someone might, for example, be worried about

- Absenteeism
- Premature retirement
- Premature death
- Health care costs

- Reduced mental performance
- Accident proneness
- Conflicts in interpersonal relationships
- Lack of concentration
- Impaired judgement
- Ineffective management and leadership
- Reduced creativity and innovation
- Slow and poor decision-making

Fig. 22   The stress iceberg

finding the money to pay a pile of domestic bills. With his mind obsessed by this problem, concentration wanders from the task in hand with the chance that a wrong button may be pushed!

An organisation's greatest asset is its employees – it is their mental as well as physical health, well-being, morale and productivity that is revealed in the balance sheets. It makes sense for companies and organisations to realise and consider that good mental and physical health is good business.

Employers can provide training and development programmes and create the right environment and atmosphere for their employees to work in the eustress zone and away from the distress zone. Ultimately, however, it is only the employees themselves who can take the steps to enter the eustress zone and keep the distress zone at bay. This involves all aspects of their lives; at home and with friends as well as at work. Identifying the sources of stress will help in taking these steps.

7 Sources of Stress

Stress is an inevitable part of our existence. Everything in our environment can be a potential source of stress but ultimately stress comes from within you; it is a result of how you perceive the situations and events in your environment. The way you perceive these situations depends to a great extent on your beliefs and attitudes. Some people have beliefs that lead them to perceive situations as threatening and challenging when in fact no real threat or challenge exists. As a result these people, called **Type As**, generate unnecessary stress for themselves. This stress can be avoided by modifying beliefs and habits. On the other hand some events during our lives will almost certainly be stressful. These are referred to as 'life events': they are mostly unavoidable and we have to adapt or readjust our lives to cope with them.

We are most likely to experience stress in our relationships with others, particularly at work and at home. Much of this stress is associated with threats and challenges to our self-esteem and self-image, the security and stability of our jobs and family relationships.

The nature of the demands

Anything in the environment that leads to activation of the stress response is termed a **stressor**. Your view of the environment and how you interact with it will determine whether or not the object or event becomes a stressor for you. However, there are some physical stressors that are clearly life-threatening and we would all see them as such. We see that we are in danger with little time to plan our action, so our alarm response is quickly summoned.

Most of us also treat novel and unusual situations as stressors, since we have no past experience in dealing with them. For these and other stressors, the amount and type of stress experienced and the activity level of the stress response depends on how we perceive the nature of the demand or threat. How important is it to us, how long does it last, how often does it occur and how clear are we about what is happening? To illustrate this, consider the 'on your marks' situation of being held up in heavy traffic.

Importance of the stressor

Some people do not mind being held up in heavy, slow-moving traffic since losing some time is of no importance to them. On the other hand others 'tear their hair out' because the delay will make them late for an important meeting. They may become angry and hostile towards other drivers, especially those jumping the queue. The point is that the importance of the stressor to you will determine the degree to which your stress response is activated.

Duration of the stressor

Being held up in a traffic jam for a few minutes may cause some irritation in a driver who is late for a meeting but if the traffic jam persists he may 'blow a fuse'. How long each stressor lasts will affect your stress balance and the extent to which your stress response is activated. Some stressors last a short time, such as a job interview, whilst others persist for long periods, for example dealing with relationship difficulties.

Intensity of the stressor

Our delayed driver will probably react less strongly to a queue of ten cars ahead than he would to a queue of a hundred cars stretching into the distance.

Frequency of the stressor

Getting out of one traffic jam only to find himself in another can keep our driver's fuse smouldering. He may meet unexpected traffic hold-ups every day whilst commuting; a car broken down, an accident or a lorry shedding its load. How often stressors occur will determine where your stress balance lies and to what extent your stress response is activated.

Uncertainty about the stressor

As our delayed driver approaches the traffic jam he may immediately treat it as a stressor because he is uncertain how long he will be delayed. 'How far does this hold-up go on for?', he mutters to himself as he views the line of traffic disappearing round the next bend. 'What will happen if I'm late for my meeting?' For many of us, worrying about what is *likely* to happen is a major source of distress.

Type A behaviour

In the mid 1950s two American cardiologists investigated the possible role of emotional stress in bringing on a heart attack. They asked several hundred industrialists and a hundred doctors treating coronary patients, 'What do you think caused the heart attack of a friend or patient?'. The majority said stress. The pressure to meet deadlines and excessive competition were singled out as the main culprits. Fascinated by the fact that emotional stress might play a role in coronary heart disease, these two cardiologists started to look at their own patients in a different way. As well as taking blood pressure and assessing cholesterol levels they looked for signs of emotional stress. It soon emerged that many of their coronary patients behaved in a similar way. Body movements and speech characteristics, as well as what the patients said during consultations, painted the same picture of individuals who were rushed, impatient, excessively competitive and ambitious and easily irritated. These early observations of what became known as Type A behaviour formed the basis of much research investigating the link between emotional stress and heart disease.

So what exactly is Type A behaviour? We described earlier how much of the way in which we interpret situations depends on our beliefs, attitudes and expectations. *Type A individuals have beliefs, attitudes and expectations that engage them in a constant struggle to gain control over their environment*. They battle vigorously to achieve and maintain control and when they sense this is being challenged or threatened, they respond by behaving in a Type A manner. Each time Type As perceive such emotional threats and challenges, *they automatically trigger their stress response*. But there is no *real* threat or challenge to their life. As a result they generate much unnecessary stress for themselves which keeps them frequently outside the normal zone of the stress balance and in the distress zone. Traffic jams, queues at the supermarket and bank, and finding the toothpaste squeezed from the middle of the tube are examples of situations that Type As find threatening. So in response to these situations their heart accelerates and pounds, their blood clots more easily and cholesterol levels rise; and all for no purpose. With his body prepared for physical action by activation of the stress response, the Type A individual can only sit and fume in his car. He cannot get out and run up and down the traffic lanes or abandon his car and run away. Nor can he engage in a fight with other motorists.

To be *Stresswise* you need to identify Type A behaviour in yourself so that you can take steps to reduce and modify it. This is possible because Type A behaviour is primarily a learned way of interacting with the environment. Type A behaviour is chiefly identified by a constant sense of time urgency and easily aroused irritation and aggravation. It is observed in an individual who tries to do more and more in less and less time, thinks about or does two or more things simultaneously, and frequently becomes angry in response to trivial happenings.

Type As might be described as agitated, hard-driving, hasty, hostile, hurried, impatient and irritable. They are often poor listeners, rushed, over-competitive and over-ambitious. People who have very few of these characteristics are described as Type B. They are calm, content, controlled, easy-going, good listeners, not easily irritated, patient and unhurried.

The assessment you completed at the beginning of this book

	NEVER	ALMOST NEVER	SOMETIMES	USUALLY	ALMOST ALWAYS	ALWAYS
Are you on time for appointments?						
Are you competitive in the games you play at home or at work?						
In conversations, do you anticipate what others are going to say (head nod, interrupt, finish sentences for them)?						
Do you feel rushed in the things you do?						
Do you get impatient in queues or traffic jams?						
Do you try to do several things at once and think about what you are going to do next?						
Do you feel you do most things fast (eating, walking, talking, driving)?						
Do you get easily irritated over trivial things?						
If you make a mistake, do you get angry with yourself?						
Do you find fault with and criticise other people?						

will give you an idea of your self-perceived level of Type A behaviour. The questionnaire on page 103 will provide a more accurate measure of this. For each question tick the box that best represents your behaviour.

SCORING

Score 5 *Always*
　　　　4 *Almost always*
　　　　3 *Usually*
　　　　2 *Sometimes*
　　　　1 *Almost never*
　　　　0 *Never*

ASSESSMENT

Add up your scores and multiply the total by 2

TYPE B	0–39	You are slightly and/or rarely impatient and aggravated. You create hardly any unnecessary stress for yourself and your health is probably unaffected.
MILD TYPE A	40–59	You are fairly and/or occasionally impatient and aggravated. You create some unnecessary stress for yourself and this may affect your health.
MODERATE TYPE A	60–79	You are very and/or often impatient and aggravated. You generate much unnecessary stress for yourself and this may affect your health.
EXTREME TYPE A	80–100	You are extremely and/or usually impatient and aggravated. You generate TOO MUCH unnecessary stress for yourself and this may affect your health.

NOTE: This is a self-assessment of your Type A behaviour. It is only as accurate as you are honest in your answers. Furthermore, Type As are often blind to their own behaviour: for example doing things fast. Type As may not think they are as fast as they actually are.

The questionnaire is based on some common Type A characteristics, many of which are easy to detect whilst others are subtle and not so obviously related to time urgency and easily aroused anger and hostility. If a person possesses a large number of Type A characteristics and displays these frequently and excessively, then he is considered to be an extreme Type A. On a scale of 0–100, the spectrum of Type A behaviour ranges from mild (score 40–59%) and moderate (score 60–79%) to severe (score 80–100%), with Type B individuals described as having very few Type A characteristics (score less than 39%). Using a similar questionnaire we have surveyed over 5000 people and found that only 10% were Type B, 80% mild–moderate Type A and 10% extreme Type A.

To help you identify Type A behaviour we will describe some typical and extreme examples.

In an attempt to gain control, Type As become 'hurry sick'; they adopt two strategies with which to save time to get more and more done in less and less time. Firstly, they practise 'speedup'; doing things fast to save time. So they eat fast, walk fast, drive fast and talk fast. Some Type As take 'speedup' to extremes. Type A men have admitted to shaving with *two* electric razors at once, to save time! On hearing this, a woman reporter admitted to us that she blow-dries her hair with *two* hairdriers at the same time. But incredible though these actions may seem to Type Bs, and also to many Type As for that matter, they are insignificant when compared to the man who liquidises all his meals so he can drink them to save time!

Not content with the amount of time saved by 'speedup', Type As turn to 'polyphasing' – doing two or more things at the same time. So they may clean their teeth or shave whilst taking a shower or continue writing a document whilst engaged in a telephone conversation on a completely different subject. As they drive to work, Type As may shave, apply make-up, eat breakfast or read the morning paper. Extreme Type As regard it as a challenge to see how many different things they can do at the same time. We heard of a businessman in San Francisco who installed a hinged desk-top in his toilet so that he could continue working whilst attending to the call of nature. By now he may well have a fax machine installed in the 'smallest room' and have acquired a head-set telephone to leave his hands free. There may be some sense in his action because many extreme Type As often ignore the calls of nature until the last minute and frequently suffer from constipation, which then makes them annoyed at the time they waste in the toilet!

Wasting time in queues is something Type As cannot tolerate. They will seek ways in which to beat, jump or avoid queueing at the bank, post office, shops, garage, traffic lights and so on. Take the supermarket situation and an extreme Type A shopper coming up to the checkouts. Whilst nobody would choose to join the longest queue, our extreme Type A shopper will make several decisions before selecting a queue. First, Type As count the number of people in the queue then multiply this by the number of items in each basket and trolley. Many of us may well do this but Type As will go further. They assess the efficiency of the checkout operator before making their choice of which queue to join. A decision is made and the 'fastest' (?) queue joined. Now, instead of simply queueing, Type As take other people as markers in other queues to see if they have made the right choice. Noradrenaline levels start to rise when our Type A realises that the markers are making better progress – 'Why do I always choose the wrong queue?', our Type A curses. Noradrenaline levels then hit the roof when the person in front of their queue holds them up by paying by credit card or cheque, and sky-high levels are reached when they get to the checkout and the till roll runs out. Our Type A finally leaves the store angry at himself and quick to vent this anger on others. Learning from this situation, Type As have adopted several strategies to beat the supermarket queue. One Type A proudly described how he took six trolleys and put five items in each and went through the express checkout six times!

The supermarket battleground may give rise to a few confrontations with other shoppers but impatience in the driving situation exposes the ugly side of extreme Type A behaviour. The typical Type A driver will always strive to drive as fast as possible, jump the red light and make a Grand Prix start just as the lights turn green. They relentlessly and obsessively drive close to the car in front and overtake at any possible, or even near-impossible, opportunity. They will compulsively switch lanes in traffic jams and take alternative routes in an attempt to avoid an apparent hold-up, often not knowing exactly where they are heading!

One extreme Type A recalled how he fought a constant stress battle always to avoid the lane which would be bottled up. 'If I see a slow-moving car or lorry I'm out of its way before I'm anywhere near it,' he exclaimed. In fact he admitted that his driving behaviour in this respect was so successful that he usually arrived early for his appointments and had to sit in his car and wait!

A participant at one of our workshops told us of his experience when being driven to a meeting by a work colleague. 'My colleague's driving was so 'Type A'. He would shout at the other drivers who got in his way, he would even wind the window down to get more effect, flash his lights and sound the horn. I swear I'm not going with him again if he drives'. A week later another meeting came up and our participant insisted that he drove instead of his Type A colleague. 'You wouldn't believe it,' he told us. 'My colleague flashed *my* lights and wound *my* windows down and *shouted at me* to do the same!'

Such driving behaviour seems harmless when compared to that of some Californian drivers who have shot dead or wounded other motorists who annoyed them! This couldn't happen in Britain . . . or could it? Recently on the M4 a driver was forced to stop, then assaulted by a motorist who had been attempting to overtake. Another motorist met his fate at the end of a tyre mallet when he angered the driver behind by allowing a woman with a pram to cross at the lights when they turned to green. Then there is the car-park space – scene of many aggressive confrontations as two drivers aim for the only vacant spot. Similar barrages of abuse fill the air when a passing place is too narrow and both drivers feel the other should reverse.

Being held up, thus having valuable time taken away from them, makes Type As angry and hostile. This reflects the general tendency for Type As to be very easily irritated and angry over trivial happenings and the mistakes of others and themselves. They can blow a fuse when they find the toothpaste squeezed from the middle of the tube if they always methodically squeeze it from the bottom. In America, we heard of a heart attack patient whose wife had put the toilet roll on the holder the wrong way round. The husband grabbed the roll, confronted his wife with it and screamed at her, 'How many times have I told you to . . .'. He had a second non-fatal heart attack. We can hear you ask yourself which way round did this man like his toilet roll? There is only one right way, as *you* know; with the paper coming over the top, of course. Well, it has to be according to the man because, 'you wouldn't see the pattern if the paper hung over the back'. That highlights another Type A characteristic – they think they are always right.

Irritation, anger and hostility generated and aimed at others harms the very person we least expect it to – ourselves. The noradrenaline released in this situation can be a killer! So the message is *do not get mad in the first place; modify your beliefs and attitudes to reduce this inappropriate Type A behaviour*. How to do this is the topic of Chapter 11.

Sometimes it is difficult to understand why such trivial things lead Type A s into the countdown for blast-off. One participant in a group that one of us (TL) has counselled for over two years would regularly recall at meetings how cutting his lawn caused him much aggravation. His wife described how she heard a noise coming from the garden and found her husband smashing the electric mower against the concrete washing-line post. With bits of mower strewn around the garden, he shouted, 'B . . . . thing kept cutting out!'. His wife pointed out that he had only bought it two weeks ago and it was still under guarantee! With such behaviour over cutting the lawn we pictured the garden as having half an acre or so of grass. It was in fact only a few square yards!

By describing Type A behaviour in this way we hope to give you a guide to identifying it in yourself and others. Type A s tend to be excessively competitive, ambitious and self-involved. They are poor listeners, interrupt whilst others are talking, head-nod to encourage the speaker to hurry along and often bring the conversation around to themselves. In conversations they frequently self-reference, that is, they often refer to themselves by regular use of pronouns 'I', 'me', 'my' and 'mine'. They frequently describe things in unnecessary detail, are obsessed with numbers and quantities and with their achievements at work and in everything they do.

We asked a Type A doctor to briefly describe her life. She replied, 'I was the youngest consultant appointed at . . . Hospital, I have a thriving private practice, have published 120 scientific articles and lectured around the world . . .'. When she had finished, we said, 'But earlier you mentioned you were married with children but you never referred to this once'. In fact, we discovered that this doctor works so much that she moved her word processor into the lounge to be with her husband.

Type A s find it difficult to believe that their way of behaving is counter-productive. Type B s give themselves more time and space to be creative and are more effective in the long run, often advancing their careers! Contrary to popular belief Type B s are also ambitious and competitive people but they go about things in a different way. As a result they achieve their goals without suffering ill health. They usually have more fulfilling family relationships and a good social life.

Type A behaviour is conducive to workaholism. Workaholics invariably suffer marital and social relationship problems, as they struggle for success and need to work longer and longer hours to achieve their goals. This clearly spells distress. You can assess whether or not you are a workaholic by completing the questionnaire below.

Your attitude to work – workaholic check list

Do you take work home most nights?

Do you frequently think about work problems at home?

Do you voluntarily work long hours?

Do work problems affect your sleeping habits?

Do your family and friends complain that you spend too little time with them?

Do you find it difficult to relax and forget work?

Do you find it difficult to say 'no' to work requests?

Do you find it difficult to delegate?

Is your self-esteem based largely on your work?

Scoring and evaluation

If you answer 'yes' to one of the above questions you may simply be dedicated to your work. However, there is a fine dividing line between dedication and obsessive devotion to work (workaholism) so be on your guard!

If you answer 'yes' to two questions you are obsessive about your work and could easily succumb to workaholism. Beware!

Answering 'yes' to three questions indicates you have an obsessive and compulsive devotion to work. The higher the score the more you are hooked into workaholism. You need to question your priorities for the sake of your marriage, social relationships, health and career. Although it may seem hard for you to believe, you can be damaging the career that you are striving obsessively to enhance.

A woman told us how her workaholic husband cancelled a week of their fortnight's family self-catering holiday because of work commitments and then described what happened. 'We set off for Cornwall via his office and waited in the car park for nearly two hours. On the Tuesday evening he said he had arranged a business appointment for the following day. He arrived back in the early hours of Thursday morning. On the way home he insisted on calling in at his office again. This time we waited just over an hour. This isn't the first time a holiday has gone like this. We are never going on holiday with him again!'

Frequently Type As find it difficult to relax and switch off from work. They are the people who come back from the Costa del Sol with three white lines across their forehead or who telephone the office every day or pack business work in their suitcase. Frequently they feel obliged to take work home and are only happy if their briefcases are bulging at the seams!

Type As will often say, 'I thrive on stress'. In fact, what they are saying is, 'I am addicted to noradrenaline'. This addiction produces a feeling of confidence and elation and often leads Type As to seek out challenging situations to keep their noradrenaline levels high.

Are you addicted to noradrenaline?

Signs of noradrenaline addiction

Mind frequently racing

Difficulty in getting to sleep

Smoking too much

Drinking too much caffeine

Hyperactive

Type A behaviour and health

Excessive, frequent and prolonged release of noradrenaline is thought to increase the risk of heart disease, high blood pressure, migraine and ulcers. Type As usually over-react to challenges and threats and, faced with a demanding situation, they over-activate their sympathetic nervous system, releasing much noradrenaline. The dangers of this were outlined in Chapter 5.

Unfortunately, self-induced stress in Type As often distorts their perception and they fail to recognise what is happening to them. However, not all Type As succumb to the ill effects of stress. It has been suggested that a personality factor described as 'hardiness' (stress resistance) interacts with Type A behaviour to minimise its risk to health. Hardy people look upon situations as challenges rather than threats. They have commitment to what they do and feel confident about gaining control. They turn stressful life events into possibilities or opportunities for personal growth and benefit. More research is needed in this area to clarify the involvement of hardiness with stress and health.

The stress generated by Type A behaviour is avoidable by modifying beliefs, attitudes and habits. This is dealt with in Chapter 11.

Life events

Some stressors are unavoidable and will affect most of us at some time during our lives. These are often referred to as **life events**, crises that must be faced: for example, illness and injury to yourself, family and friends, and bereavements. Other crises may occur, such as marital disharmony, problems with children, financial difficulties and work problems. There are also events that require some adjustment on our part, such as moving to a new house, changing jobs, children starting school. Our stress response is activated to help us deal with these changes, events and crises. However, research has shown that if we experience too many life events during a short period, our adaptive and coping resources may be overtaxed and this can lead to ill health.

Researchers in the United States asked several hundred people which events that occurred during their life required the most readjustment. Forty three life events were selected as being the most common and stressful; these are shown in the table on page 112. You will notice that some events, such as

LIFE EVENTS: check your score and assess your risk

Death of partner	100
Divorce	73
Separation from partner	65
Jail sentence	63
Death of close family member	63
Injury or illness to yourself	53
Marriage – your own	50
Given the sack at work	47
Reconciliation with partner	45
Retirement	45
Ill health in member of family	44
Pregnancy – your own	40
Sexual problems/difficulties	39
Addition of new family member	39
Major business or work changes	39
Change in your financial state	38
Death of friend	37
Change to a different type of work	36
More arguments with partner	35
Take on a large mortgage	31
Mortgage or loan foreclosed	30
Change in responsibilities at work	29
Child leaves home	29
Trouble with in-laws	29
Outstanding personal achievement	28
Wife begins or stops work	26
Child begins or ends school	26
Change in living conditions	25
Change of personal habits	24
Trouble with boss or employer	23
Change in working hours or conditions	20
Change in residence	20
Child changes schools	20
Change in church activities	19
Change in social activities	18
Change in sleeping habits	16
Change in number of family get-togethers	15
Change in eating habits	15
Holiday	13
Christmas (coming soon)	12
Minor violations of the law	11

This scale is adapted from Holmes and Rahe's Life Change Index; Journal of Psychosomatic Research, 1967, Vol. 11, pp. 213–218.

illness and bereavement, are traumatic and likely to give rise to distress whereas others, such as marriage, birth of a child or moving house, might be expected to be pleasant and enjoyable experiences. However, they all require a change in the person's life to readjust to the new situation. You will see that each event is given a score on a scale from 0 to 100. The scores are based on how much adjustment people felt they needed to make in order to cope with each situation, if getting married is rated at 50 points. As expected, most people rated death of a spouse at the maximum score of 100 whilst at the other end of the scale, Christmas was valued at 12 and minor violations of the law 11. Subsequent research using this scale showed that those people who scored over 100 points in their previous year had an increased risk of suffering a major illness during the next two years (see p. 128).

Even though these types of stressors are unavoidable, our beliefs and attitudes can play a major part in how we perceive them and how much stress, if any, we experience. For example, bereavement is undoubtedly a major stressor but our religious beliefs may reduce the stress experienced.

Family, social and work situations

We spend about a third of our life at work, a further third sleeping and the remaining third with our family and friends. Many people find that the most distress in their lives arises from relationships with others, both in the family and social setting, and at work. Look back at the life events list and you will see how many are associated with relationships; for example marital disharmony, problems with children, problems with neighbours, problems with the boss or co-workers. Similarly, there are a number of events relating to work. Work is commonly cited as a major cause of distress and there are many reasons for this, for example:

- Work overload – simply having too much to do.
- Time pressures and impossible deadlines to meet.
- How well and to what extent you feel your skills and abilities are being used.
- Poorly defined or understood job role.

- Changes in procedures.
- Poor communication – not knowing what is going on and not feeling a part of the organisation.

Sometimes these demands may be imposed on you by others and you feel pressured and not in control. Use the checklist opposite to assess your level of job satisfaction. Being dissatisfied with a particular aspect of your job may not mean you find it stressful so you should also rate your perceived stress experience for each item.

There is no scoring system for this checklist but carrying out this exercise will help you to focus on those aspects at work which may be sources of stress for you. This is a first step for dealing with stress at work. Using the coping strategies described in Part Three, you should be able to find ways of resolving any problems.

Work stress can also be self-imposed: for example, setting unrealistic goals, attempting to change too much too quickly. You may need to stand back and ask yourself how your stress is arising. Are you asking too much of people who work for you? Are you creating unnecessary stress for yourself? Are you a workaholic?

It may be that you regard your stress as being derived only from work or home but usually it is from both. Stress from family arguments or financial worries can affect our work performance; our minds might not be on the job in hand and accidents or mistakes can easily occur. Feeling generally distressed will make us less able to handle the inevitable pressures and demands of our job. On the other hand, a happy home life with few major worries can help us ride through the pressures of work without distress. Similarly, a day at work full of pressure, demands and situations that lower our self-esteem can continue when we get home. Then it takes just a minor irritation to make us snap at our partner or shout at the children.

Often before we realise what is happening, we can enter into a vicious circle and things can go from bad to worse. So stress must be tackled throughout all aspects of our life. This is what the *Stresswise* programme is about; learning to deal with stress and to care for yourself and your relationships. We should remember that family, social and work situations can be a source of much joy, love, support and stimulation. They can provide security and self-esteem. Building on these can keep you away from the distress zone and direct you into the eustress zone.

IDENTIFYING STRESS AT WORK		
Tick any aspect of your job with which you are dissatisfied. Also, for each aspect write the number which best represents your view of how much stress you experience.		
Stress rating		
0 = no stress at all　　　　3 = very stressful 1 = slightly stressful　　　4 = extremely stressful 2 = moderately stressful		
ASPECTS OF YOUR JOB	DISSATISFIED	STRESS RATING
The physical conditions at work, e.g. ventilation, noise, lighting, heating		
The freedom to choose your work		
The freedom to get on with your work		
Your colleagues		
The recognition you get for good work		
Having more than one immediate boss		
The amount of responsibility you are given		
Your rate of pay		
Your opportunity to use your abilities		
Industrial relations between management and workers in your organisation		
Your chance of promotion		
The way your organisation is managed		
The attention paid to suggestions you make		
The number of hours worked		
The amount of variety in your job		
The security of your employment		

PART THREE

Dealing with Stress

To deal with stress effectively you must adjust your stress balance to keep it in and around the normal zone. This means not going too far and too often into the distress zone and making it easier to enter and remain in the eustress zone when the need arises. Getting the right balance is simply a question of adjusting the weight in the pans. Clearly there are two ways in which this can be achieved; either by altering demands or by improving coping ability (Figure 23).

Having read Parts One and Two of *Stresswise* you now know one of the most important ways of dealing with stress – **being aware of it**. You will now know what is happening in your body when your stress response is activated. You should now be able to recognise physical and mental signs of overactivation of the stress response. You should have some insight into how this can affect your health and performance. Furthermore, you should be able to identify personal sources of stress.

You are now in a position to think about your own stress and learn how you can manage stress effectively. There are many different strategies for doing this. Those described here are the ones we have found most useful and effective in teaching our groups and individuals. We have chosen to present these strategies in five chapters. There is inevitably much overlap between the contents of each and because of this, there is some repetition of information and advice. However, we feel this will serve to emphasise the importance of the issues we describe, their relationships with one another and the holistic approach we advocate for dealing with stress.

To help you learn and practise the skills for dealing with stress, we have provided a *Stresswise* kit containing biodots, self-adhesive hearts and a plastic heart paperclip. Biodots are devices which monitor the level of activation of the stress response and are used to help you learn to relax. The self-adhesive hearts and the clip are cueing devices. These are simply to remind you to practise the actions we advise you to follow for dealing with distress. We explain how and when these can be used at appropriate points throughout the text.

Getting the right balance

When the balance tips into the distress zone (perceived demands outweigh perceived ability to cope), adjustments can be

BEING STRESSWISE MEANS GOING FROM THIS . . . . . .

TOO MANY DEMANDS

- Too many life events
- Unable to delegate
- Perfectionism
- Poorly organised
- Not able to prioritise
- Unrealistic expectations
- Poor time management
- Unsuitable job
- Never seek help
- Can never say 'no'

POOR COPING RESOURCES

- Low love and support
- Type A behaviour
- Unable to relax
- Do not smile or laugh
- No sense of humour
- Not assertive
- Low self-esteem
- Negative thinking
- Unaware of signs/symptoms of stress—stress concept
- Inadequate sleep/rest
- Drink too much caffeine
- Drink too much alcohol
- Poor state of health
- Unbalanced and poor diet
- Smoke too much
- Unfit—lack of exercise

..... TO THIS

- Keep count of life events
- Can say 'no'
- Organised
- Prioritise
- Realistic expectations
- Avoid perfectionism
- Able to delegate
- Seek help when necessary
- Good time management
- Avoid uncertainty
- Suitable job

REDUCING DEMANDS

- Awareness of stress concept
- Can recognise signs and symptoms of stress
- Able to relax – practise relaxation technique
- High love and support
- Good state of health
- High/secure self-esteem
- Low type A behaviour
- Healthy balanced diet
- Low/moderate alcohol and caffeine consumption
- Reduce/stop smoking
- Exercise regularly-fit
- Smile and laugh
- Good sense of humour
- Positive thinker
- Assertive

GOOD COPING RESOURCES

Fig. 23 Factors altering demands and ability to cope

Fig. 24   Getting the right balance; reducing demands

made to reduce demands (Figure 24) or to build up coping resources so that the balance swings back into the normal zone.

We will inevitably encounter situations in which demands outweigh our ability to cope. No matter how much our coping resources are increased, demands have the potential of being one step ahead. For example, it is certain that we will be confronted by novel situations as part of daily living. Furthermore, from time to time our ability to cope can be reduced by changes in our general state of health, allowing demands to get

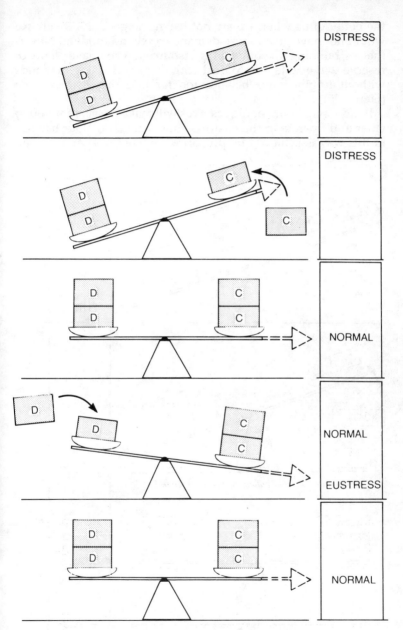

Fig. 25 Getting the right balance; building up coping resources

the better of us when we are not feeling so good. Normally we would not have given these demands a second thought. Nevertheless, building up your coping resources so you have plenty of reserve will enable you to deal with extra and taxing demands without tipping your balance too far into the distress zone (Figure 25).

Building up your coping reserves will make it easier for you to enter and operate in the eustress zone. Adjusting your balance in this way is achieved by preparing yourself to keep one step

Fig. 26   Getting the right balance; increasing demands

ahead of 'reasonable' demands by learning the skills to build up your coping resources. For most of the time this will keep you in the normal zone but with a season ticket to enter the eustress zone. However, additional and excessive demands will inevitably arise and tax our ability to cope. So increasing your coping reserves will help lessen the blow and keep you away from the depths of the distress zone; avoiding the bad and ugly!

Ironically, under some circumstances, thinking we have too much ability to cope can also cause distress. This can occur in two ways. Firstly, when the perceived demands may be too few and consequently do not balance our perceived ability to cope. We can feel under-used. We feel we have the ability to do more and our skills and expertise are not being utilised. Clearly, it is not appropriate to say to someone in this situation,'Go away and reduce your coping reserves to match your level of demand'. The right balance is achieved by increasing demands (Figure 26).

Secondly, if we have unrealistic views of our abilities to handle demands, we may perceive that we can cope with more and more when in fact we cannot. To avoid tipping the balance into the distress zone we must be realistic about our expectations thus reviewing our ability to cope.

Adjusting the balance is a continuous operation of altering demands and coping resources. You are the only person who can adjust your stress balance. Keeping your balance right can be achieved by learning the skills to reduce or increase demands and by building up coping resources.

8 *Altering Demands*

REDUCING DEMANDS

- KEEP COUNT OF LIFE EVENTS
- LEARN TO SAY 'NO'
- ORGANISE YOUR LIFE
- WORK OUT YOUR PRIORITIES
- BE REALISTIC ABOUT WHAT YOU CAN ACHIEVE
- AVOID PERFECTIONISM
- DELEGATE
- SEEK HELP WHEN THE GOING GETS TOUGH
- FIND A JOB WHICH SUITS YOUR PERSONALITY AND ABILITIES
- LEARN TO WORK EFFECTIVELY
- AVOID UNCERTAINTY

INCREASING DEMANDS

- TAKE UP A HOBBY OR PASTIME
- JOIN AN EVENING CLASS
- JOIN A VOLUNTARY OR COMMUNITY ORGANISATION
- REAPPRAISE YOUR JOB/JOB ROLE

Reducing demands

Keep count of life events

Too many changes in a relatively short period can tax your ability to adapt, resulting in distress and ill health. To avoid this problem, always keep an eye on your number of life change events. Use the life events scale on page 112 as a checklist and keep a tally of your score.

Try to prevent too many of these events occurring in a short time. So, for example, if you have just changed jobs, moved house to an area miles from your family and friends and taken on a large mortgage, it would be wise to postpone other plans or projects until you have settled. If you are nearing retirement, consider making a gradual rather than sudden change from full-time work to full retirement.

Traumatic life events, such as divorce, serious illness or death of a loved one, will most likely reduce your coping reserves. This will make you more vulnerable to the dangers of distress. At such times it would be wise to consider the number of demands you are dealing with and to build up your coping reserves through love and support (see page 191).

The life events list is by no means exhaustive. You should identify events in your life which require an adjustment in order for you to handle them. These can be pleasant as well as unpleasant events. Give each a score according to your judgement of how they compare with the events and scores shown on the life events scale.

For each and every one of us, there is a 1 in 10 chance (10% risk) that we will suffer a serious illness during the next year. But your life events score during the previous year may increase your risk of ill health during the following two years (see table below). So scoring 150 to 299 points will increase your chance to about 1 in 2 (50% risk). This may be a result of excessive cortisol release since many life events require attention over a relatively long period. Under these circumstances, cortisol can reduce our ability to fight infection and makes us more susceptible to disease.

Note that the life events scale is based on studies of many thousands of people. Having a risk of 1 in 2 means that, of 100

SCORE	RISK OF ILLNESS DURING NEXT TWO YEARS
300 or more 150–299 100–149	80% 50% 30%
less than 100	no change in risk

people scoring between 150 and 299, 50 would become ill within 2 years. So this scale is not very accurate in predicting the illness vulnerability of individuals. This is because each of us will perceive the events differently and the ability to cope with them will vary considerably from individual to individual. Nonetheless, it is wise to consider the effects on our health and performance of accumulating stressors.

Learn to say 'no'

Some people find it very difficult to say 'no' to requests from friends and work colleagues even though they feel unable to cope with more work. They often feel it is a sign of uncooperation or an admission that they cannot handle more work. They feel that refusing to help may prejudice their promotion prospects or affect their relationship with others.

More work here does not just mean work connected with our jobs but also requests to join another fund-raising event, coach the local football team, service the car, decorate the house and so on. As the saying goes, 'If you want something done always ask a busy person', because they are usually the ones who are unable to say 'no'!

If you feel you cannot take on more work then be honest, clear and assertive in your reply. Point out how much work you are currently doing and what is waiting to be done, or that there are circumstances in your domestic life making it difficult for you to work extra hours.

It is important that you say 'no' in the right way. Julie, a secretary, told us of her main source of stress at work. 'My boss always gives me a pile of work at around 4.00pm and expects it to be completed before I finish work at 5.00pm. Sometimes I'm still typing at 6.00pm.' We asked why she had never said anything. 'I'm afraid he will think I'm not being cooperative and I might lose my job.'

We pointed out the consequences of her distress and suggested she asked her boss to prioritise the work in the following way. 'I realise that this work is important; however, I finish work at 5 o'clock and when you give me work at this time of the day I'm usually here until 6. I have an important appointment tonight so I would appreciate it if you would kindly sort out those items that are urgent and I'll make sure they are done before I leave. I will come in early tomorrow morning and deal with the rest.'

So what happened when Julie tried this way of saying, 'No, I'm not prepared to tackle all those demands'? Mr Smith did just as she asked. In fact, he designated only two letters as urgent. Julie left work at 5 o'clock and tells us that she has only worked later than that on two occasions since. Julie's response was assertive. She stated her case clearly and honestly, was firm and polite and suggested what might be done to help resolve the situation. Being assertive will help you say 'no' in the right way (see page 195).

Whatever the situation or circumstance, one thing is certain; if you take on more than you feel able to handle then you are likely to feel pressured, harassed and rushed, and your performance will suffer. Jobs will take longer to do and may not be done well. So saying 'no' and seeking clarification of priorities, planning ahead and being realistic about what you can achieve makes sense in the long run.

Organise your life, prioritise and be realistic about what you can achieve

Some people find it helpful to plan ahead: from day to day, week to week, month to month and year to year. Others have the philosophy of 'live for today' which reminds us not to be too obsessed with rigidly organising the future. However, even carefree people must plan ahead in some way or another. This should include setting priorities and being realistic about what can be achieved.

Setting realistic goals

Many unnecessary demands can result from setting unrealistic goals which are difficult to attain. This is particularly true for Type As. Being realistic about what you can achieve will reduce demands. This will mean being honest about your abilities. Winning promotion to a job you have always wanted but find you cannot handle is one of the major sources of distress.

To set your priorities and realistic goals, take a piece of paper and write your objectives and goals in life. Use the headings of

SELF   FAMILY   FRIENDS   WORK

Write everything down, even those things you feel are impossible to achieve. Here are a few suggestions to help you.

SELF

- stop smoking
- need more exercise
- need to lose weight
- need time to relax

- what would I do if I had more time?
- what do I enjoy doing?
- learn a new skill or subject
- would like to travel more

FAMILY AND FRIENDS

- spend more time with them
- visit relatives more often
- like a different house or new car
- help children more with school work/projects

- take trips out together
- need to make new friends

WORK

- type of work
- commuting distance
- shiftwork and working away from home
- work abroad

- ambitions
- start own business

Now, for each one identify the importance you attach to it. Grade the importance by using five stars for top priority and one star for the least. Now go through the list again and mark those items that you feel you can realistically achieve with an R or highlighter pen. Delete those which you feel are too difficult to attain or are unattainable. Now sit back and review your list. You may need to decide on a time-scale for some items; what are your goals for the next month, year and so on. Construct a short-term and long-term plan. You will probably realise that many of your goals are achievable simply through minor changes in your lifestyle, perhaps by devoting a little more time to one area rather than another.

By undertaking this exercise you are planning your life,

prioritising your activities and being realistic about what you might achieve. In this way you will have more chance of fulfilling your expectations. When expectations are achieved self-esteem is high and this will enable you to deal more effectively with stress. Frequent failure to achieve unrealistic goals severely damages self-esteem and opens the door for aggression or depression.

Clearly circumstances change, so you will need to update your lifeplan regularly, maybe weekly or monthly. You may find it an interesting exercise to construct your lifeplan at this stage of the book and again when you have finished reading it.

Organising and prioritising

Planning and prioritising your work can help you reduce and avoid distress. Much anxiety can build up if the tasks that need to be completed seem never-ending. We start to wonder how and when to fit in other essential activities. Look at your work schedule, prioritise and plan the order of completion, considering deadlines and importance. It is not much use spending a lot of time and effort on minor tasks, and perhaps getting tired and irritated, when more important and urgent jobs need to be completed, and done well. Try to concentrate on one task at a time, particularly if this is a major and important one.

One man described to us how he dealt with his office letters, memos, reports and so on. 'I start reading a document on the top of the pile of papers on my desk. I get half way through and my mind wanders to a letter I caught a glimpse of half way down the pile. I can't resist leaving the document I'm reading to pull out the letter. I start reading the letter, think "Yes I must do this, that or the other" and then push it to one side. I go back to the first document and, having lost my train of thought, I start at the beginning. Soon I'm off into the pile again. As a result I don't seem to get things done very quickly and end up thinking and worrying about several things at the same time!'

Our advice to this man was to prioritise: sort quickly through your papers and put them in order of importance. Make three piles and colour-code them; very urgent (green – go), urgent (amber – get ready) and not urgent (red – stop). Work through each pile in turn, dealing with the very urgent before proceeding to the urgent and so on. Of course, priorities can change so the order should not be considered fixed.

Wading through a sea of paper is one of today's worst office stressors. You can check your efficiency and your need to prioritise by ticking the corner of a document each time you read or look at it. You may be surprised at the number of ticks some documents accumulate.

Keeping a diary and appointment book is a very effective way of organising yourself. Write as much information as is appropriate about appointments, deadlines and reminders as they arise, for both work and homelife. You will need a large enough diary to provide the space for notes and suggestions and drawing up plans for the day and week but this does not mean buying an additional briefcase to hold your 'mega-diary'! In this way you will have less need to make notes on scraps of paper which may get lost. Everything is in one place and time is not wasted wading through piles of notes. Give a high priority to personal and domestic problems since failure to deal with these will inevitably affect your work.

A well-maintained diary will help to reduce the worry and anxiety of wondering if you will remember all your appointments. Make time every day to work with your diary. Use self-adhesive coloured dots or highlighter pens to prioritise tasks. Keep to the same colour for a specific activity: red for deadlines, green for meetings, yellow for telephone calls, for instance.

Avoid creating unnecessary deadlines and cluttering up your calendar with appointments. Use the heart paperclip to mark the day of the week in your diary. This will serve as a reminder that ignoring the effects of excessive demands can be costly to both your health and work performance.

An important factor in planning and setting priorities is being realistic about what can be achieved. If you are asked to give a time for completion of a task, do not put yourself under unnecessary pressure by saying next week (just to make yourself look efficient) when you know you may not meet that deadline.

Avoid perfectionism

Perfectionists in particular need to be realistic. Type As are bugged by perfectionism. Always striving obsessively to achieve perfection is usually counter-productive. Many perfectionists believe that if perfection is not achieved, disaster is bound to result. It must be realised that the 'perfect and best' result can only be achieved once in a lifetime. Striving to better your best performance each time leads to unnecessary demands, pressures, distress and feelings of failure if it is not achieved. Settle for your best effort and be content with what you have done. You probably will have produced a good and satisfactory job without ending up distressed.

Perfectionism as described here should not be confused with working conscientiously and diligently to achieve your best performance and good results, particularly where it is essential for tasks to be done correctly. So getting rid of perfectionism does not mean attending less to your work and making mistakes or producing a poor performance. We describe perfectionists as those people who are obsessive about producing a 100%, absolutely correct piece of work in everything they do.

Why do perfectionists strive for perfection? We asked a self-confessed perfectionist to tell us about the advantages of perfectionism. She said, 'It sometimes produces an excellent piece of work which pleases me very much.' Are there any disadvantages, we asked? She thought for a while and replied, 'Yes I suppose there are. I often worry about not doing a good job. This means I usually stick to techniques I know well so I hardly ever experiment with new ideas. I am self-critical, set myself high standards, get very upset if things are not turning out the way I want them to. Sometimes I spend such an incredible amount of time trying to produce a perfect result that I become agitated. Usually I end up settling for what I had achieved in the first place. In the meantime, I waste a lot of time and feel annoyed with myself.'

Another key factor in planning and prioritising is managing time. Learning the skills to manage your time effectively can reduce demands and increase coping ability, thus helping tip your stress balance into the eustress zone. Some aspects of time management are dealt with in the section on modifying and reducing Type A behaviour (see page 179).

Delegate

Another way of reducing demands at home and work is to delegate. If you are in a position to delegate at work then you have undoubtedly demonstrated that you are good at your job and you are probably managing, supervising and directing others. There can be a tendency for you to believe (particularly if you are a Type A) that jobs will get done better and quicker if you do them all yourself, but this is often not the case. You can become overloaded with tasks which could be delegated to someone else.

When you delegate, make sure you choose the person best suited to the job and who has the time to devote to it. Give clear instructions and information on what you expect and reassure the person of your confidence in them and that you will be available should they need any advice or assistance.

There are many positive benefits to delegating. Giving responsibility to another person makes them feel part of what is going on, that you have confidence and trust in them and it provides them with the experience they will need for their career advancement. Their self-esteem is boosted and they will probably perform well with their stress balance in the eustress zone.

Women often face a mountain of demands due to their multiple roles; looking after the home and family as mother, meal planner, shopper, cook, cleaner, laundress and so on. This job is frequently combined with employment outside the home. Clearly, reducing demands by delegating domestic duties can help avoid distress.

Seek help when the going gets tough

Seeking help and support from others in the tasks you perform can be mutually beneficial in reducing workload and demands. Rather than struggle, ask for help. Struggling on your own can be very distressful and this will certainly make a task more difficult to complete. It is better to admit you need help and then satisfactorily complete the task than to struggle to produce a poor piece of work, or even fail.

Find a job which suits your personality and abilities

If you are looking for a job, you should seek one which you feel suits your personality, skills and ability. If you are already in a stressful job then review the demands placed upon you and your abilities to handle them. Consider your work expectations and be realistic about your ability to achieve them.

Learn to work effectively

Many aspects of your work may be decided by your employer or organisation, leaving you with little control over what you do. In situations where this is distressful, stand back and ask yourself whether the demands and pressures are real and reasonable or whether your perceived lack of control is simply a result of your unrealistic expectations.

Clearly, the physical conditions of your work environment are important, not least from a safety point of view: bad lighting, insufficient heating, poor ventilation, noise, overcrowding, lack of privacy and uncomfortable office furniture are frequent sources of dissatisfaction, frustration and distress. Many employers appreciate that the right physical environment will encourage productivity and creativity, so you should not be hesitant about approaching your employer if you feel these things are causing you distress. There are some changes you can probably make for yourself such as brightening your immediate work area with coloured posters, postcards, photographs, cartoons and plants.

There is much that you can do to organise your work. Take short breaks from routine tasks even if it means simply closing your eyes for a few minutes and relaxing. Practise a relaxation technique (such as those described in Chapter 9) at your desk or bench. Arrange your office or surroundings so you have to get up and walk to the filing cabinet or to answer the telephone. When you talk on the telephone concentrate on the task in hand and do not polyphase (do more than one thing at a time). Be assertive, say 'no' when you feel overloaded with work. Seek immediate clarification about what is required from you when you are asked to do a job. At this stage you should point out any difficulties or problems you foresee and ask for help if necessary. It is always more difficult to do this after the event, though you can always go back and ask again. In the meantime, you may have worried unnecessarily over any difficulties and problems.

If you have a lot to do, arrange your jobs in order of priority. It is usually most productive, effective and satisfying to complete one job at a time before moving on to the next.

Do not rush; spend some time thinking about how to tackle problems and plan your course of action. Routine jobs are often best tackled using a strict timetable such as opening mail first thing in the morning. Do not clutter your diary with appointments or make appointments when you know you may not be able or will be pushed to keep them. Leave some time for yourself during the day for relaxation and never miss your lunch and tea breaks. Use them effectively: get out of the work environment, go for a walk or relax and read a novel. Learn to manage your time effectively.

Most people work with others, so you should pay particular attention to giving and receiving support and building self-esteem with respect to your work. Learn the art of good communication and assertiveness. Develop the art of listening – you will not only learn more by listening rather than talking but you will form better relationships – people like to talk and tell you about themselves. Control your voice in discussions; do not become threatening or emotional. You will get your views over better by using clearly stated points in an assertive manner. Do not underestimate the value of good humour.

Avoid uncertainty

Uncertainty is the cause of much distress. Worrying about what might happen if . . . may be unnecessary. Find out the facts about things before you get anxious and panic. When you have collected as much information as you can, it might then be obvious that your initial fears and worries were ill-founded and you will have avoided unnecessary distress. On the other hand, if your worries were warranted you will be prepared and can plan all the possible alternatives and seek help if necessary. This will make you feel less uncertain. Coping with demands and pressures is easier if you know exactly what you are dealing with.

Increasing demands

There are a number of situations where an individual may feel that there are too few demands in their life: too little stimulation and not enough challenges. They feel they have the capability to handle more. They may feel under-used, bored and frustrated. Self-esteem suffers, motivation declines and eventually performance becomes poor in all they do.

One such situation where this may arise is retirement. This involves a sudden change from active and busy full-time work to a less demanding life with few deadlines to keep. As a retired person, you can experience an overnight change from being an important part of an organisation and making a valuable contribution to society, to a position where your usefulness within society seems diminished. It is not possible to reduce your perceived coping ability to match your lower perceived demands, so you should take on new demands. Maybe take up a hobby, join an evening class and learn something that you always wanted to do but never had the time for whilst working. Plan and do the things you did not have the time for, such as taking a long trip abroad. Keep up and renew friendships, become involved in community projects, local clubs and voluntary organisations. Plan your day as if it were a working day; build in time for domestic duties, shopping, walking, hobbies and so on. But beware – do not increase demands to the point where your stress balance tips into the distress zone.

Another situation where too few demands lead to distress is where an employee feels their abilities and skills are not adequately used. The simple remedy is to ask the employer for more work. On the other hand, it may be that someone in this position is in the wrong job. Finding the right job to suit your aptitude and abilities perfectly is not an easy task. Where there is a significant mismatch, distress inevitably results. Correcting this situation may mean requesting the organisation to re-appraise job role with a view to moving you to a different job or it may mean leaving the job and seeking one which is more suitable.

We can find ourself in a position of having too few demands if we lose our job, face a change in family situations when children leave home or our partner dies. When we get back on our feet it may be necessary to increase demands in a similar way to the retirement situation described above.

9 Learning to Relax to Increase Coping Resources

- MAKE TIME FOR YOURSELF TO RECHARGE YOUR BATTERIES
- DEVELOP RELAXING DAILY ACTIVITIES
- BREATHE CORRECTLY
- USE BIOFEEDBACK
- PRACTISE PROGRESSIVE AND DEEP MUSCULAR RELAXATION
- PRACTISE MEDITATION

Recharge your batteries

A period of relaxation is a time to recharge your batteries. It is a period of minimal sympathetic nervous system activity which allows the parasympathetic nervous system to increase its influence on body function. When you are relaxed your noradrenaline, adrenaline and cortisol levels are low and your body activity opposite to that experienced during the activation of the stress response. Heart rate and breathing decrease and the body feels warm due to dilation of the blood vessels. Sweating decreases, saliva secretion increases, muscle tension decreases, and the mind feels settled. However, your body is always ready to respond to danger within a split second even from a deep state of relaxation.

Develop relaxing daily activities

There are a number of specific procedures that bring about a

state of relaxation, for example yoga, meditation, progressive and deep muscular relaxation, autogenics, self-hypnosis and biofeedback. Many of these procedures must be learnt and practised regularly. They should become as much a part of your life as brushing your teeth, and not restricted to when you are feeling or expect to feel stressed. Learning these techniques takes time and you should not expect too much too soon. Furthermore, it can take a while before the benefits are experienced but the results are worth waiting for. Later we describe the techniques we use and take you through the procedures so you can learn to achieve a state of relaxation.

There are also a number of activities that can be built into your daily routine to make you feel relaxed and revitalised. Simply taking a hot bubble bath, floating in a swimming pool, taking a steam bath, sauna or jacuzzi can bring about a state of relaxation. So too can going for a pleasant walk, taking a weekend break away from home, listening to your favourite music (baroque music appears particularly effective), reading your favourite books, a night out at the theatre, an evening meal at your favourite restaurant.

Massage is a particularly effective way of relaxing the muscles which in turn leads to a calm mind. Also taking up a hobby, a leisure activity, joining a club, tinkering with the car, tackling a DIY project or developing new interests can all be relaxing as long as they are looked on as relaxation activities. But beware; some of these activities can be stressful if tackled in the wrong way.

A well-planned holiday of at least a week's duration is a good way to recharge your batteries. However, take heed, even a holiday can be packed full of distress. There might be airport delays, language and currency problems, the hotel and resort do not come up to your expectations and there is plenty of rain instead of 'guaranteed' sun. Stomach trouble strikes, you get sunburnt, and your partner forgot to pack your favourite beachwear. What is intended to be a relaxing holiday can turn into a distressful nightmare! Preparation and planning can help avoid many of these problems and minimise distress.

Relaxation should not be regarded as something done only outside work. Taking your regular coffee and lunch breaks is important; these are times for you to recharge your batteries. Try to get away from your office or work surroundings. Go for a short walk or read a favourite book. If you feel stressed during the day, sit back for a few minutes and practise a quick relaxation technique. Try the quieting reflex (QR). It takes only a few seconds and with practice achieves a body state opposite to activation of the alarm reaction.

QR

STEP ONE: Close your eyes. Pinpoint in your mind what is annoying or stressing you.

STEP TWO: Say to yourself, 'Alert mind, calm body. I'm not going to let this get to me.'

STEP THREE: Smile to yourself. You can practise smiling to yourself without showing a smile on your face. In this way your smile will not be obvious to others around you.

STEP FOUR: Breathe in to the count of three while imagining that the air comes in through holes in your feet. Feel the sensation of warmth and heaviness flowing throughout your body, starting at your feet and ending at your head.

STEP FIVE: Breathe out to the count of three. Visualise your breath passing through your body from your head and out through the holes in your feet. Feel the warmth and heaviness flow through your body. Let your muscles relax, let the jaw, tongue and shoulders go limp.

Now open your eyes and resume your normal activity.

With practice over several months, QR becomes automatic. It provides a pause for you to decide whether or not to stay stressed, tense and annoyed or to shift into a less irritated and more relaxed state.

Are you breathing correctly?

This may seem a silly question; how, people ask, can an everyday automatic activity like breathing be carried out incorrectly? This is more of a problem than you may imagine. Incorrect breathing can cause much discomfort, ill health and a feeling of distress. A part of our stress response is to change

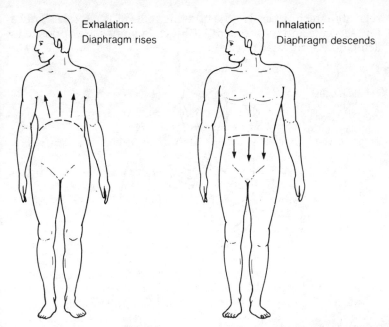

Fig. 27 Movement of the diaphragm during correct breathing when at rest

breathing patterns. During physical exertion, breathing rate and depth increase, because we need to take in more oxygen to eliminate the vast amount of carbon dioxide produced by muscle activity. The chest moves outwards and upwards to allow more air into the lungs. When we breathe at rest, it is movements of the diaphragm that exchange the air in our lungs. As the diaphragm moves up and down, the abdomen moves in and out but the chest remains almost stationary (Figure 27).

In emotional stress, activation of the stress response leads to rapid and deep breathing. The upper part of the chest is mainly used for this type of breathing. With no physical outlet for our stress response, such breathing (called **hyperventilation**) flushes too much carbon dioxide out of the lungs, making the blood and tissues more alkaline.

In some situations breathing can become rapid and very shallow from the chest. Insufficient air is taken in and out of the lungs to flush out the accumulating carbon dioxide so it builds up in the blood, making it more acidic. These patterns of

Hand on chest should be almost stationary (should not rise or fall) as you breathe in and out

Hand on abdomen should move outward as you breathe in and inward as you breathe out

Fig. 28   Are you breathing correctly?

breathing which make the blood too acid or too alkaline can result in abnormal body functions.

Our breathing pattern can reveal our emotions. Anxious people breathe rapidly and talk as they breathe in (inhale). On the other hand, depressed people sigh frequently and talk as they breathe out (exhale). If people remain in a state of high sympathetic arousal and anxiety for a long period, their breathing pattern at rest and during moderate activity can alter. Over time their breathing shifts more from diaphragmatic movement to chest movement.

So, are you breathing correctly? Try this simple test. Lie on your back in a comfortable position, support your head on a pillow and relax. Place one hand on your abdomen and the other on your chest (Figure 28). As you inhale and exhale note the movement of your abdomen and chest. If you are breathing correctly the hand on your abdomen should rise as you breathe in and fall as you breathe out. Your chest should not be moving so the hand on your chest should not rise or fall as you breathe. So, if the hand on your chest is moving and the hand on your abdomen is stationary then you are breathing *incorrectly*.

Procedure for correcting your breathing and using deep breathing for relaxation

Lie on the floor on your back. Support your head on a pillow. Bend your knees, keeping your feet flat on the floor. Place one hand on your chest and one hand on your abdomen. Breathe slowly through your nose. Keep your mouth closed. Take slow gentle deep breaths. As you *inhale* push your abdomen out against your hand – feel your abdomen expand and your hand rise. Hold for two seconds* and then *exhale* slowly through your nose. Feel your stomach deflate and your hand fall. Repeat four times.

When you have mastered this exercise, follow the same procedure in the sitting and standing positions. Eventually, you can do the exercise without positioning your hands on your chest and abdomen. Concentrating on your abdominal movements in this way will slowly help to correct faulty breathing patterns. The procedure can be used as a relaxation technique in its own right, when you feel tense and anxious. It is a useful quick method that can be applied almost anywhere – sitting at your desk, in a stationary car, on a train or bus.

Correct breathing and the deep breathing technique are used in most other forms of relaxation such as the two we describe below. So before attempting these, practise the breathing exercise.

Use biofeedback

Progressive and deep muscular relaxation and meditation are recognised, well-tried techniques which we recommend and use in our workshops, training and counselling programmes.

---

*Sufferers from respiratory complaints including asthma and bronchitis may find breath-holding uncomfortable or difficult. These sufferers should avoid long breath-holding in this exercise and others described later. Stop the breathing exercise if you feel light-headed at any time during the procedure and resume your usual pattern of breathing until you feel able to continue.

When we teach these procedures we use biofeedback devices, such as biodots, to enable the person to monitor their level of relaxation. So before we take you through the progressive and deep muscular relaxation techniques we will describe biofeedback and the use of biodots.

What is biofeedback?

Biofeedback is the use of instruments and devices to enable a person to monitor body responses triggered during the stress response such as heart rate, blood pressure, muscle tenseness, skin temperature, sweating and brain electrical activity. The technique allows the user to see for themselves their level of stress response activation and state of relaxation. Biofeedback is a useful tool for relaxation training, as it will indicate to the user whether or not a state of relaxation has been achieved.

One of the most commonly used methods involves measuring the amount of sweat on the skin. During the stress response sweating increases; in the relaxation response it decreases. The amount of sweat on the skin is detected by two small metal plates (electrodes), each strapped to a finger. A small safe electric current is passed across the electrodes. When the skin is moist, due to the presence of sweat, the current passes easily over the skin. When the skin is drier, the passage of the current is impeded because skin resistance is higher. So this technique measures the skin resistance and is known as the galvanic skin response or GSR. In fact, GSR techniques form the basis of lie detector apparatus. Usually when a person lies, their emotions trigger the stress response, leading to sweating.

For biofeedback information, the skin resistance is converted into a sound. Increased stress and tension lead to a high-pitched sound, relaxation results in a lowering of the sound.

Skin resistance meters are relatively inexpensive devices suitable for self-help purposes. More sophisticated and expensive equipment is needed to obtain biofeedback from other body activities such as brain wave activity. However, a very simple and inexpensive device for self-help is the biodot. We have included these in your own *Stresswise* kit.

What are biodots?

Biodots are small self-adhesive temperature-sensitive discs that can be stuck to the skin. They indicate changes in skin temperature by changing colour (see colour interpretation chart on the back cover of this book).

How do biodots monitor stress?

Remember what you learnt about the stress response and skin temperature. Biodots monitor skin temperature changes caused by differences in the amount of blood flowing through the skin. More blood flow – skin is warmer; less blood flow – skin is cooler. When a person is tense and stressed blood vessels constrict, reducing skin blood flow, thus lowering the temperature of the skin. The biodot will appear yellow, amber or black. When a person is calm and relaxed blood vessels dilate, increasing skin blood flow, and this raises the temperature of the skin. The biodot will appear green, turquoise, blue or violet.

How to use biodots

Stick the biodot where it will be easily seen but not easily dislodged. Recommended sites are on the inner surface of the wrist, and the base of the thumb and forefinger (see Figure 29). If care is taken the biodot can remain attached to the wrist or hand for several hours.

Fig. 29   Biodot positions

Other factors affecting biodot colour

It is important to remember that certain conditions and activities apart from your level of stress response activation will affect biodot colour changes. These include:

• **Ambient temperature**   If the external temperature is cool or cold the skin blood vessels constrict (biodot colour in black/amber/yellow range). If it is warm or hot the skin blood vessels dilate (biodot colour in green/blue/violet range). When you have acclimatised to the prevailing temperature any change in colour will indicate a change in the level of stress.

• **Exercise**   Colours indicating high stress levels will be observed when you are taking moderate exercise and going about your daily activities, even though you may not be emotionally stressed or tense. This is because the skin blood vessels constrict during exercise, allowing more blood to flow to the muscles. In severe exercise, when the body is hot, the skin blood vessels will dilate allowing heat to be lost.

• **Alcohol consumption and smoking**   Alcohol dilates blood vessels and the biodot will show green, blue or violet. Smoking causes constriction of the blood vessels and the biodot may appear black, amber or yellow.

Biodots – an aid to relaxation

Biodots are particularly useful as biofeedback aids during relaxation training, motivating the user and providing reassurance that they have achieved relaxation and stress reduction. Use them when you try the progressive or deep muscular relaxation and meditation methods described below.

Additional supplies of biodots can be obtained from *Stresswise* (see page 200).

Progressive and deep muscular relaxation

In this technique each of the main groups of muscles is tensed then relaxed in sequence, hence the name progressive muscular relaxation (PMR). At each stage the mind is concentrated first on the feelings of tension and then on relaxation. With practice, you can learn to be aware of muscle tenseness so you can easily and automatically convert tension into relaxation. For example, many drivers find their shoulders hunched and hands gripping the steering wheel so tightly that the knuckles turn white. Through PMR, you will recognise this tension and automatically relax the muscles, thus reducing head, neck, shoulder and back pains and stiffness.

When the body muscles are relaxed, the mind relaxes and this reduces sympathetic nerve activity, leading to a decrease in heart rate and blood pressure. However, the technique is not recommended for sufferers of high blood pressure (hypertension). This is because the tensing of muscles causes elevation of the blood pressure which then decreases when the muscles are relaxed. So if you suffer from hypertension it is wise not to increase your blood pressure further by tensing the muscles during PMR. Instead we advise you to practise deep muscular relaxation (DMR). This technique is similar to PMR but the muscles are not deliberately tensed prior to relaxing (page 152).

You will need to find a suitable place to practise these techniques; somewhere quiet and warm, where you will not be disturbed. It is advisable not to try them for up to two hours after eating a heavy meal, and use a firm, upright chair rather than an armchair, which can encourage drowsiness. It is helpful to get someone to read the procedure to you so you can concentrate on the movements and technique. Alternatively, ask someone with a soft relaxing voice to tape-record the instructions (we have deliberately written them almost as a commentary) and play the tape back to yourself. A pre-recorded audio-cassette of these procedures is available from *Stresswise* (see page 200).

Procedure for progressive muscular relaxation

Allow 15 minutes

Warning: Do not over-tense or over-stretch your muscles. Stop if you feel uncomfortable or experience any pain. Sufferers from high blood pressure are advised to practise deep muscular relaxation (see page 152) instead of using PMR.

Place a biodot on your hand and note the colour. Sit comfortably well back in the chair so your back is supported and both feet rest flat on the floor a little way apart. Rest your arms in your lap. Keep your head straight with your chin parallel to the floor. Your breathing should be abdominal and relaxed – gentle, slow and unforced.

Close your eyes and direct your attention to each part of your body in turn. As you tense each set of muscles, concentrate on the tenseness and tightness (hold the position for five seconds or so) and then as you relax the muscles, concentrate on the sensation of relaxation. Notice how the tenseness disappears and the muscles feel at ease, warm and heavy (stay in this position for about ten seconds).

Shrug your shoulders towards your ears; pull them up as far as you can; feel the tenseness in your shoulders and neck. Hold for five seconds. Now relax; feel the muscles relax. Relax for ten seconds.

Now pull your shoulders down towards the floor. Concentrate on the tenseness. Hold for five seconds and relax for ten seconds.

(Always hold the tenseness for about five seconds and the relaxation for about ten seconds.)

Bend your right arm and make your bicep muscle stand out as much as you can; tense the muscle, hold it . . . now lower the arm and relax. Turn the palm of your right hand upwards. Clench your fist as firmly as you can. Concentrate on the tenseness and relax, unfolding your fist. Now stretch your fingers out as far as they will go, feel your fingers stiffen and the thumb pushing away from the fingers. Hold it, feel the tenseness and relax; feel the fingers curl gently inwards.

Bend your left arm and make your bicep muscle stand out; tense the muscle, feel the tenseness: lower the arm and relax. Turn the palm of your left hand upwards. Clench your fist as firmly as you can and concentrate on the tenseness. Hold it . . . now unfold your fist and relax. Stretch your fingers as far as they will go. Feel the fingers stiffen, the thumb pushing away from the fingers. Hold it . . . now relax and notice the fingers curl gently inwards.

Concentrate on your legs. Straighten your right leg and push your foot away from you; feel the tenseness of the muscles on the front of your thigh. Point your toes as far away as you can, now bend your foot back at the ankle. Feel the muscles tense in your right calf. Hold it . . . and relax. Tighten the muscles in your right foot. Curl your toes and when your foot feels as tense as you can make it . . . relax.

Straighten your left leg and push your foot away from you; feel the tightness of the muscles at the front of your thigh. Point your toes as far away as you can, now bend your foot back at the ankle. Feel the muscles tense in your left calf. Hold it . . . and relax.

Tighten the muscles in your left foot. Curl your toes and when your foot feels as tense as you can make it – relax. Relax.

Now lift yourself up by tensing your buttock muscles. Lift higher and higher – hold it . . . now let the muscles relax.

Contract your abdominal wall muscles – make your waist as small as you can. Feel the tenseness. Hold it . . . and relax.

Now turn your attention to your head. Move your head gently forward until you feel the muscles in your neck and back tighten. Hold it and then return your head back to the centre and relax. Tilt your head to the right, feel the tenseness in your muscles and then return your head to the centre and relax. Now tilt your head to the left, feel the tenseness and return your head to the centre and relax.

Now clench your teeth tightly – feel the pressure and tenseness of your jaw muscles. Allow your jaw to sag slightly, feel the muscle tenseness ease. Let your mouth drop open and feel the tenseness ease further . . . and relax. Now close your mouth and push your tongue against the roof of your mouth – feel the tenseness and pressure . . . now relax the tongue behind the lower teeth. Relax.

Smile broadly – feel the change in muscle tenseness – hold it . . . and relax. Screw up your eyes, tighter and tighter. Hold it . . . and relax them back into the sockets. Now pull your eyebrows down, now raise them as high as you can, hold it . . . and relax. Relax.

Concentrate on your breathing: feel your abdominal muscles move slowly out and up as you breathe in and then down and inward as you breathe out. Your breathing should be slow, gentle and shallow.

Now quieten your mind. Allow your thoughts to drift through your head, without trying to pursue them. As easily as thoughts come into your mind they leave, and as easily as they leave more thoughts effortlessly come in. Recall happy memories. Picture a walk along the seashore: the waves, warm water lapping around your feet as they sink in the sand. Sun glistening on the water. Deep blue cloudless sky. The cries of the seagulls.

Sit quietly for five minutes and enjoy the state of relaxation you have created throughout your body. Your body should feel warm and heavy – totally relaxed. Look at your biodot. If you are more relaxed than when you started PMR your dot colour should be more towards the blue end of the scale.

Before you stand up, gently stretch your body and take two or three deep breaths.

Procedure for deep muscular relaxation

Allow 15 minutes

Place a biodot on your hand and note the colour. Sit comfortably well back in the chair so your back is supported and both feet rest flat on the floor a little way apart. Rest your arms in your lap. Keep your head straight with your chin parallel to the floor. Your breathing should be abdominal and relaxed – gentle, slow and unforced.

Close your eyes and direct your attention to each part of your body in turn. Each time, relax the muscles and concentrate on the sensation of relaxation. Notice how the tenseness disappears and the muscles feel at ease, warm and heavy (stay in this position for about ten seconds).

Concentrate first on your left leg. Focus your attention on each part of your leg in turn, starting at your toes and working toward your hip. As you relax each set of muscles, feel the tension drain away and notice the sensation of limpness, heaviness and warmth. Relax your toes . . . concentrate for about five seconds on the feeling of relaxation (do this between relaxing each part). Now relax the instep . . . heel . . . and ankle. Now relax your calf muscles . . . feel them become limp, heavy and warm. Now relax your knee . . . thigh . . . and your hip. Concentrate on the relaxation of your left leg . . . heavy, limp and warm.

Now focus your attention on your right leg. Concentrate on each part of your leg in turn, starting at your toes and working towards your hip. As you relax each set of muscles, feel the tension drain away and notice the sensation of limpness, heaviness and warmth. Relax your toes . . . concentrate for about five seconds on the feeling of relaxation . . . now relax the instep . . . heel . . . and ankle. Now relax your calf muscles . . . feel them become limp, heavy and warm . . . now relax your knee . . . thigh

... and your hip. Concentrate on the relaxation of your right leg ... heavy, limp and warm.

Now concentrate on your left arm. Focus your attention on each part of your arm in turn, starting at your fingers and working towards your shoulder. Relax your fingers and thumb ... feel them curl inwards ... relax your palm ... now your wrist ... forearm ... elbow ... upper arm ... and lastly your shoulder. Concentrate on the limp, heavy and warm sensation.

Now concentrate on your right arm. Focus your attention on each part of your arm in turn, starting at your fingers and working toward your shoulder. Relax your fingers and thumb ... feel them curl inwards ... relax your palm ... now your wrist ... forearm ... elbow ... upper arm ... and lastly your shoulder. Concentrate on the limp, heavy and warm sensation.

Now concentrate on your stomach muscles. Let them relax ... limp, heavy and warm.

Now concentrate on the base of your spine. Slowly work your way up the spine towards the neck, relaxing each part of the spine and associated back muscles as you progress towards the neck. Feel the muscles relax, becoming limp and heavy as your back sinks into the chair ...

Now relax your shoulders again ... feel them drop towards the floor, limp, heavy and warm ...

Relax your neck muscles but keep your head straight, your chin parallel to the floor. Your head should now be balanced on your spine.

Now focus your attention on your head. Relax your jaw, let it drop and feel your mouth slightly open ... relax your tongue and feel it drop behind your lower teeth ... relax the muscles around your eyes ... feel them become limp, heavy and warm ... relax your forehead ... and scalp. Your head should feel totally relaxed, heavy and warm.

Concentrate on your breathing: feel your abdominal muscles move slowly out and up as you breathe in and then down and inward as you breathe out. Your breathing should be slow and gentle.

Now quieten your mind. Allow your thoughts to drift through your head, without trying to pursue them. As easily as thoughts come into your mind they leave, and as easily as they leave more thoughts effortlessly come in. Recall happy memories. Picture a walk along the seashore: the waves, warm water lapping around your feet as they sink in the sand. Sun glistening on the water. Deep blue cloudless sky. The cries of the seagulls.

Sit quietly for five minutes and enjoy the state of relaxation you have created throughout your body. Your body should feel warm and heavy – totally relaxed. Look at your biodot. If you are more relaxed than when you started DMR, your dot colour should be more towards the blue end of the scale.

Meditation

Whereas PMR and DMR concentrate on muscle relaxation, meditation concentrates on relaxing the mind. The technique is very simple. The mind is focused for twenty minutes on a word or sound, known as a **focal device**. This is repeated over and over again in the mind. As the technique is performed, thoughts will pass in and out of the mind. When the mind wanders it can be brought back to the focal device. With practice the mind will wander less often and this allows the repetition of the word to engage the left side of the brain in a meaningless task. This side of the brain deals more with logical and analytical thinking and normally dominates our consciousness (Figure 30). When the word is repeated over and over again the left brain is occupied in the monotonous task of attending to the repetitious information. As this happens, the activity of the right side of the brain takes over. This side of the brain is involved with intuition, imagination and creativity. Suppressing the analytical activity of the left brain and allowing intuitive dominance of the right brain results in a reduction in stress response activation and an increase in tranquillity; a feeling of serenity.

During meditation, the body's oxygen requirement drops, the heart and breathing slow, blood pressure decreases. In fact, a general state of relaxation is achieved. Recordings of brain wave activity show more alpha rhythms which are characteristic of a state of relaxation.

There is a variety of meditation methods, but the basic technique is a very effective and beneficial relaxation tool which

Left
Logical
Analytical
Scientific
Rational

Right
Intuitive
Artistic
Imaginative
Creative

Fig. 30   The left and right hemispheres of the brain

can be used by everyone. The meditation procedure we describe below uses a word as the focal device. Like PMR and DMR, meditation can be undertaken anywhere reasonably quiet, warm and free of possible distractions. It may not be suitable for those suffering from epilepsy and some psychiatric disorders.

Procedure for meditation

Allow 20 minutes

Find a quiet, warm place where you will not be disturbed. Sit in a comfortable upright position, place a biodot on your hand and note the colour. Make a note of the time. Breathing should be slow, gentle and abdominal. Close your eyes then repeat aloud the word 'om' or 'one'. Do this several times then repeat the word more quietly and then quieter still until you are not moving your lips but merely thinking the word over and over in your mind. Do not concentrate on keeping the word in the forefront of your mind – it should not be like counting sheep. You will find that your mind begins to wander. Thoughts will come into your mind; 'I've got to buy some postage stamps on the way home', 'I must book the car in for a service'.

Let thoughts wander into your mind and then let them leave by simply thinking the sound over and over again. (The sound of the word is purely a means of helping you clear your mind.) Continue in this manner for 20 minutes, then stop and sit quietly for a minute or so. Gradually and slowly open your eyes. Note the colour of the biodot.

You are looking for a change in the colour of your biodot

towards the turquoise blue range, to show that you have achieved a state of calm and relaxation and reduced your level of stress. Look for the signs of relaxation such as warm hands and feet, and salivation.

End your relaxation by gently stretching your arms and legs and taking two or three slow deep breaths.

Do not use an alarm to tell you when the 20 minutes is up – open your eyes slowly and look at a clock when you feel that 20 minutes has passed. With practice you will find it easy to judge 20 minutes. The time will pass very quickly. Sometimes you will find it hard to believe you have sat and relaxed for 20 minutes. After practising meditation regularly, twice a day for about two to three months, you may experience periods of deep mental relaxation.

Try to meditate regularly each morning and evening at a time when your home or office is reasonably quiet. Take precautions so you will not be disturbed. While you are learning the technique, you may find it helpful to use earplugs (available from chemists). Unplug the telephone and ensure the room temperature is comfortable. Avoid eating for about two hours beforehand. Late evening meditation may affect your sleep since meditation usually increases alertness.

We recommend you practise PMR, DMR and meditation in the sitting position without supporting the head. If you are lying down, with head supported in a relaxed state, it is easy to fall asleep. The aim of practising a relaxation technique is to achieve a state of physical and mental calmness different from sleep.

Relaxation techniques must be learnt and you should not expect instant success. With the aid of biodots you will be able to monitor your progress and the effects of the technique. Eventually, you should be able to take a short meditation or muscular relaxation any time and anywhere.

The benefits of relaxation

The reduction in sympathetic nervous system activity brought about by relaxation techniques has the benefit of allowing the body to rest and recharge its batteries. Your coping abilities usually increase, making it likely that you will experience eustress rather than distress. However, there are a number of other benefits. Some doctors now use relaxation methods, particularly PMR, DMR and meditation, to treat patients with high blood pressure and high blood cholesterol, sometimes without the use of medication. In the same way that blood pressure and cholesterol levels rise as sympathetic arousal increases, so levels drop when sympathetic activity declines. Patients practising relaxation for one month or more have shown a decrease in blood cholesterol and other blood fats.

It has been reported that regular meditators make fewer visits to their doctors than non-meditators and that a variety of physical ailments can be alleviated through meditation. While teaching relaxation techniques, we have seen some remarkable changes in our students. A 38-year-old woman with Raynaud's disease (painful cold fingers due to constriction of the digital arteries) reported that the condition disappeared two weeks after she learned to meditate. Three years later, she has not experienced the symptoms again. We have taught many people with sleep problems to meditate. In most cases their problems have disappeared within a week or two of starting meditation. A woman on tranquillisers managed to reduce her dose under the supervision of her doctor after we taught her to meditate. It must be said that these problems might have disappeared anyway or that it was not the meditation itself but the care and attention given to these people that did the trick. Maybe so, we cannot prove otherwise, but there is enough evidence to support the belief that the biological consequences of meditation can bring about such changes. A number of studies and surveys also support this view.

Other benefits of relaxation, and particularly of meditation, are increased mental alertness, improved concentration, creativity and memory, leading to better performance and enhanced or improved relationships. Regular practice can lead to improved well-being and a different, more rational attitude and view on life.

10 Reviewing Lifestyle to Increase Coping Resources

REVIEW YOUR

- DIET
- CAFFEINE CONSUMPTION
- ALCOHOL CONSUMPTION
- SMOKING HABITS
- FITNESS AND EXERCISE
- BODY WEIGHT
- SLEEP AND REST

There are a number of ways in which you can alter your lifestyle to build up your resistance to stress. If you are healthy and fit you will feel good about yourself: your self-esteem will be high, and your irritability, anger and hostility levels low. The following lifestyle review looks at diet, use of stimulants (caffeine and nicotine), alcohol consumption, body weight, fitness and exercise, sleep and rest. It is not a comprehensive guide to health and fitness but deals with some aspects which we feel are particularly relevant to the stress response and its activation and which we use regularly in our workshops.

Diet

- EAT A WELL-BALANCED DIET
- WATCH YOUR FAT INTAKE
- CHECK YOUR FIBRE INTAKE
- MAKE SURE YOUR MINERAL, VITAMIN C AND B COMPLEX INTAKE IS ADEQUATE
- DRINK TWO PINTS OF WATER EACH DAY
- EAT BREAKFAST

We have all been inundated with advice on what to eat and what not to eat, so much so that many people find it confusing and stressful. We hear, 'Eat this, don't eat that, eat more of this and less of that'. One minute we are told, 'Eat this', the next, 'Don't'.

Despite the massive amount of research into how our diet affects our health and what is a healthy diet, there is still much that is not understood. For example, the link between dietary fat intake and heart disease is far from clear. But the message we are given makes it sound so simple and clear-cut. 'Large amounts of fat in our diet increase blood cholesterol. High blood cholesterol is associated with heart disease.' The latter point is known to be true but is high blood cholesterol related so conclusively, as we are led to believe, to what we eat? The relationship between diet and blood cholesterol is controversial and extremely complex and the arguments for and against this issue are outside the scope of this book.

So what should we do? It is a question of being sensible about our diet. Eating an excess of anything will cause problems and a little bit of what you fancy will probably do you no harm. To become obsessive about what you eat can cause much distress and feelings of guilt. This could do more harm than the so-called unhealthy diet itself. Of course there are those, such as angina sufferers and heart attack victims, who may need to regulate their diet but for most of us such strict rules may not be appropriate. However, everyone can benefit by taking the *stress* out of *eating*.

One of the main aims of the fight and flight reaction is to provide a quick and plentiful supply of energy for muscle activity by mobilising fats and glucose stores. The level of blood fats, including cholesterol, and the level of blood glucose increase. During the alarm reaction, the levels of cholesterol and triacylglycerol (another type of fat) rise far more than they can from dietary sources. In fact, only about 10% of our cholesterol comes from the diet; the rest is made by the body. We described earlier how levels of blood cholesterol rise during periods of stress. We used the example of tax accountants meeting deadlines to complete their clients' tax returns. Try to remember this point when you feel pressured because if you are stressed you will have higher levels of cholesterol circulating in your blood than normal.

Remember also that increased blood cholesterol and fat levels are associated with coronary heart disease and increased susceptibility to blood clot formation. For angina sufferers and heart attack victims, one high-fat meal can lead to red cell sludging which can block the fine coronary blood vessels. The result could be a heart attack which may be fatal.

It is therefore wise to reduce your intake of fat, particularly saturated fat, so when your blood fat and cholesterol levels rise during stressful periods, there is less chance of them reaching potentially harmful peaks. Eating high-fat meals whilst you are under pressure and feeling stressed is therefore not to be recommended.

Another way of reducing blood fat is to eat more fibre. It works like this. Fats stick to the fibre, which is not absorbed by the body so the amount of fat absorbed is also reduced. Be careful not to eat too much fibre (the recommended daily intake is 30 grams) because certain vitamins and minerals can also attach to fibre, so less of these will be absorbed into the body.

It is also advisable to make sure you have enough vitamin B complex (comprising several different vitamins) and vitamin C in your diet, particularly when you feel pressured and stressed. These vitamins are required for a number of vital body processes. Vitamin C is required for fighting infections and wound healing, and vitamin B complex for good mental activity and many of the body's chemical processes. They are also needed to make the hormones used during the stress response, and there is some evidence suggesting that inadequate vitamin C levels may encourage the accumulation of cholesterol in arteries. Foods rich in vitamin C are blackcurrants, rosehips, citrus fruits, leafy green vegetables such as Brussels sprouts and cabbage. Vitamins of the B complex are found in a variety of foods; rich sources are wholegrain cereals, yeast and meat.

A well-balanced diet should provide an adequate amount of vitamin C and B complex; however, to ensure you are not lacking these two vitamins when under stress, we advise you to take supplements. A vitamin C supplement of up to 400mg/day is adequate; taking over this amount for months at a time could cause kidney stones. Take vitamin B complex according to the Recommended Daily Allowance (RDA) shown on the package.

Your mineral and trace element intake should also be adequate. Although a well-balanced diet should contain essential nutrients in the correct proportions, look particularly at your intake of calcium (good food sources are dairy produce and spinach), magnesium (nuts, cereal grains and fish), iron (red meat and offal, green leafy vegetables and wholegrain cereals), zinc (bran, meat and dairy produce), manganese (wholegrain cereals, nuts and avocado pear), selenium (meat, dairy produce, wholegrain cereals) and chromium (wholegrain cereals, brewer's yeast and cheese). All these minerals are involved in the stress response and deficiencies caused by their depletion during periods of stress can lead to poor body functioning and ill-health.

This is not to say that you should increase your food intake when under stress. Rather, by eating a balanced diet in the first place, you ensure that your body is prepared to deal with increased pressure when the need arises. Similarly, protein levels can decrease during periods of stress; an action of cortisol is to mobilise body proteins for energy. So attention should be given to a balanced protein intake during periods of prolonged stress. This is important because when we feel distressed we often do not feel like food, at the very time we should be taking extra care about eating properly.

It is not advisable to take megadoses of vitamin supplements except under medical supervision. Subjected to excessive doses, the body can become saturated with the vitamin or mineral and this may hinder or prevent vital body functions. Taking supplements according to Recommended Daily Allowances will do no harm (RDAs are usually shown on the label of the container).

Increased sweating during the stress response can lead to dehydration. Drinking one to two pints of water each day will help prevent this and stop the blood from thickening too much. Thick blood clots more easily.

As well as taking the above precautions, it makes sense to eat a balanced diet; that is, a diet which has both the right number of calories to provide sufficient energy and the right proportions of all essential nutrients. Such a diet comprises about 10–15% protein, 30–35% fat (made up of half saturated and half unsaturated, that is polyunsaturated and mono-unsaturated), 50–60% carbohydrate and adequate vitamins, minerals and water.

For the average person this may mean:

- cutting down on fat intake (particularly saturated fats – these are mainly animal fats)
- increasing the amount of complex carbohydrate eaten to increase fibre intake (wholegrain cereals, wholemeal, bran, pulses, nuts and seeds) and

- eating more fruit and vegetables, preferably fresh or frozen, not tinned.

Eating sensibly is not simply a question of eating the right amounts of food but also adopting a sensible eating pattern. It is very easy to miss meals when under pressure. Breakfast can become one cup of coffee and lunch a quick sandwich as you work. On the other hand, life can become one continuous meal when under stress.

Let your body tell you when to eat. Keeping to the traditional '3 meals a day' rule is not always necessary. It is often better to eat smaller, more frequent meals spaced throughout the day instead of eating one or two very large meals. In this way the digestive system does not work 'overtime'.

Breakfast is considered by nutritionists to be the most important meal of the day – it gets us off to a good start. Skipping breakfast leads to mid-morning tiredness, irritability, depression, confusion and an inability to concentrate. Ideally, breakfast should contain unrefined carbohydrates, protein and some fat, for example porridge, low-fat yoghurt, low-fat sausages or fresh fruit. This provides a steady level of blood sugar throughout the morning. Lunch should be a top-up meal, and the evening meal the lightest of the day. It is better to eat your evening meal early because the digestive processes may cause sleeplessness. Eating a light evening meal will give your digestive system a rest overnight.

The type of foods we eat can also affect our mental activities. What we eat as well as when we eat can affect our memory and ability to concentrate. Meals excessively high in carbohydrates and low in protein make it less easy for people, particularly those over 40 years old, to concentrate and deal with mental tasks.

Caffeine

> ● REDUCE CAFFEINE INTAKE
> ● SWITCH TO A DECAFFEINATED DRINK

Caffeine is found mainly in coffee, tea, cocoa, drinking chocolate, chocolates and cola drinks.

Caffeine content of some common beverages in milligrams

		Amount (mg)/cup
Coffee	filter	240
	percolated	192
	instant	104
	decaffeinated	3
Tea	brewed	75
	instant	35
Colas		30–65
Cocoa		5–145
Chocolate		20

Note: these figures are approximate. Actual quantities of caffeine per cup depend on the brand and strength of drink prepared.

Excessive caffeine consumption (about 1000 milligrams of caffeine each day, equivalent to 6 cups of coffee) is considered harmful. Caffeine stimulates the nervous system and production of the catecholamines, particularly noradrenaline. It makes sense not to produce more noradrenaline than you need for the activities you are undertaking. Taking an excessive amount of caffeine is like being in a state of high arousal with your stress reaction operating at full stretch.

Caffeine, through the effects of noradrenaline, increases alertness and performance, but many people find that too much of it during the late evening can lead to sleep disturbances. High caffeine consumers may be simply addicted to the stimulating effect and pleasant feeling induced by noradrenaline.

Caffeine increases heart rate. Add this effect to the increased heart rate caused by the catecholamines released during stress response activation and you can end up with problems. Such increases in heart rate lead to increased heart workload and can be a danger for those with coronary heart disease. More seriously, caffeine can stimulate the heart to beat irregularly and this can lead to fatal rhythms.

Caffeine also stimulates the production of acid by the stomach. This can cause heartburn, indigestion, and aggravate ulcers. Since the stomach reduces its activity during the stress response, caffeine taken at this time will stay in the stomach longer and have more time to exert its potentially harmful effect. Other digestive tract problems such as colitis and piles can also be aggravated by caffeine.

There is also evidence suggesting that high caffeine intake can lead to increased blood cholesterol through the action of noradrenaline. Four cups of caffeinated coffee can increase cholesterol in the blood by 5% and ten cups by around 12%. Such increases, added to the rise in cholesterol during periods of stress, as well as that obtained from the diet, may elevate blood cholesterol to potentially harmful levels.

So cut down on the amount of caffeine you drink. Try switching to decaffeinated coffee and herbal teas and other caffeine-free drinks.

Alcohol consumption

> ● KEEP ALCOHOL CONSUMPTION WITHIN THE
> RECOMMENDED LIMITS
> ● AVOID DRINKING SPREES
> ● TRY SWITCHING TO LOW-ALCOHOL DRINKS AND
> MINERAL WATER

Most people have experienced the effects of alcohol. One or two drinks can be relaxing; three or four and the party takes off! You soon forget your worries. This is the problem; alcohol helps us to forget our distress so when under stress some people turn to alcohol to solve their problems. Usually they drink more and more, only to find that when they have sobered up their problems are still there. Unfortunately many people turn to alcohol for its tranquillising effect. This is clearly not the answer to dealing with problems.

Excessive alcohol consumption can become a health problem leading to a number of physical and behavioural disorders but many experts believe low quantities of alcohol may have some benefits. The situation is far from clear.

What is an excessive alcohol intake? For simplicity, alcohol intake is measured in standard units. One standard unit is half a pint of beer or lager, one glass of wine, a small glass of sherry, a measure of vermouth, a single measure of spirits. The recommended sensible limit of alcohol intake for men is 21 units each week and for women 14 units. (This amount should be spread throughout the week and not concentrated into one or two days.) A person with this level of intake would be considered a light drinker. Moderate and excessive weekly limits are shown in the table below.

	MEN	WOMEN
Low (Light drinkers)	1–21	1–14
Moderate (Moderate drinkers)	22–35	15–21
Excessive (Heavy drinkers)	Over 36	Over 22

Like stress, alcohol affects the heart and blood vessels. Low to moderate amounts of alcohol could be beneficial but in excess it is certainly harmful, particularly for heart disease sufferers. Alcohol causes blood vessels to relax, leading to an increase in blood flow – a fact that has led to the view that a 'wee tot of whisky' will improve the circulation. This relaxing action of alcohol on the skin blood vessels will make a person feel warmer. You can see this by checking the colour of your biodot before and after a drink. A word of warning here for the elderly. A small drink only at bedtime makes you feel warm and relaxed and will aid sleep but make sure you are tucked up in bed before you take your drink. If you do not, the dilation of your skin blood vessels means you will lose body heat quickly and this could lead to **hypothermia** in inadequately heated rooms.

Excessive amounts of alcohol consumed over a long period can cause abnormally high blood pressure, particularly in those who have a family history of hypertension. For this reason hypertensives should limit their alcohol consumption. Drinking sprees can give rise to abnormal heart rhythms which can be fatal, particularly in those with diagnosed coronary heart disease. This is thought to be due to an alcohol-induced action of the catecholamines, which we know cause cardiac arrhythmias. Another reason for not blowing a fuse when you have been drinking.

Alcohol also affects the blood fat levels. First the good news. It appears that HDL-cholesterol ('good' cholesterol) increases with high alcohol consumption. This is clearly beneficial but now the bad news; excessive alcohol consumption causes an increase in blood tr (fat) levels.

It is the liver that is involved in the breakdown of alcohol and whilst it is doing so it cannot attend very well to blood sugar and fat. So fats from the diet tend to remain in the blood rather than be taken up and dealt with by the liver. This results in high blood fat levels which make the blood more viscous, increasing the risk of clot formation and red-cell sludging. Heart disease sufferers should keep their alcohol intake low and seek the advice of their doctor on the subject of alcohol consumption.

It must also be remembered that alcohol is highly calorific and can lead to weight problems and poor nutrition. One standard unit contains about 8 g alcohol, providing 56 calories of energy. This is the equivalent of 3 teaspoons of refined sugar! If you are overweight then think twice before drinking alcohol. Whilst a small amount of alcohol stimulates the appetite, heavy drinkers may loose interest in food. This often leads to poor nutrition and deficiency of vital vitamins and minerals.

Alcohol can destroy self-esteem, family relationships and careers. It can also interfere with sleep and rest, two of the main allies we have for dealing with stress. Alcohol depresses brain function. This leads to impaired judgement and co-ordination thus reducing performance and increasing the likelihood of accidents.

All this adds up to the conclusion that a little of what you fancy (but only a glass or two) may be good for you but too much is certainly not, and stress and heart disease definitely do not mix with alcohol. So keep track of your daily and weekly alcohol consumption and stay within the recommended limits. Try switching to low-alcohol, low-calorie drinks and mineral waters.

Smoking

- REDUCE OR STOP SMOKING
- AVOID PASSIVE SMOKING

It is not the purpose here to enter into the 'whether or not to smoke' debate. There is, however, much medical evidence associating smoking with a number of diseases including lung cancer, heart disease and circulatory problems. Many smoking-related diseases are also cited as being stress-related, so it makes sense not to smoke.

However, some people smoke to cope with their demands and pressures. Simply having a cigarette in their hand can lower reaction to potential stressors which would otherwise cause distress. Who is to say which is worst for these people – the harmful effects of smoking or those of stress? We recommend using healthy coping strategies (as we describe in *Stresswise*), rather than an unhealthy (smoking) coping strategy. Research evidence indicates that smoking together with potential stressors can lead to a stress response activation higher than the effects produced by either smoking or stress alone. One reason for this may be that, during the stress response, breathing is more rapid and deeper, thereby allowing more cigarette smoke to enter the lungs than during more relaxed conditions.

Nicotine is the main culprit as far as the stress response is concerned. Again, like caffeine, nicotine stimulates the production of the catecholamines, particularly noradrenaline. This may be a reason why smokers tend to have lower levels of vitamin C in their body (vitamin C is used in the production of stress hormones). As we pointed out earlier, lack of vitamin C may cause the deposition of cholesterol in the arteries and could be part of the reason why smoking is linked to coronary heart disease.

It has been suggested that smokers simply smoke to maintain high levels of noradrenaline which stimulate the pleasure centres of the brain. Noradrenaline addiction again? Nicotine also stimulates the heart, increasing its rate, and the blood vessels, causing them to constrict. Both these effects can exacerbate heart and circulatory disease problems: coronary heart disease, hypertension and intermittent claudication (cramps in the legs due to poor circulation).

It is not only nicotine that is to blame. Carbon monoxide in cigarette smoke combines with the oxygen-carrying haemoglobin in the red blood cells, reducing the blood's oxygen levels. Both carbon monoxide and nicotine cause the blood to clot more easily.

For some people there can be some beneficial effects of smoking. Nicotine, through the effects of noradrenaline, increases alertness and good performance, benefits associated with the fight aspect of the alarm reaction. However, smokers are not usually fighting or exercising, so the benefits of nicotine are not used in an appropriate way.

Recently, much evidence has accumulated to suggest that breathing other people's cigarette smoke, known as passive smoking, can be harmful to health. So where possible, avoid passive smoking. At times this may mean asking someone not to smoke and doing this assertively will avoid unnecessary distress that can easily arise in such situations.

Fitness and exercise

> - USE THE STAIRS, NOT THE LIFT
> - WALK ALL OR SOME OF THE WAY TO WORK
> - EXERCISE EVERY DAY
> - LEARN TO EXERCISE WHILE YOU ARE WAITING

The alarm reaction was designed for fighting or running away: in other words, for increased activity. When we exercise, essentially the same alarm response is put into action but without the accompanying emotions. For our ancestors and grandparents, life was far more physical; pulling ploughs and walking miles used up the higher circulating blood fats and catecholamines produced by their stress response. Today, it is up and down escalators and lifts and using the car for the shortest of trips. We live in an age of inactivity. Studies have shown that our schoolchildren are the unfittest they have ever been. One man said to us that the PMR programme was the most exercise he had taken for years! It is also an age of psychological stressors and emotional crises. These trigger our stress response, preparing us for action when in fact little muscular activity takes place. However, because of our generally sedentary lifestyles there is a reluctance and sometimes little opportunity to burn off the action of the catecholamines. Arguing on the telephone switches on the alarm reaction but we are sitting motionless – apart from maybe pounding the desk. So, the actions preparing us for fight or flight are not used. We put the telephone down and are left with high circulating blood fats and glucose and blood that will clot more easily. The best way to get rid of these is to exercise. Take a brisk walk at lunchtime or after work. If you are upset at the office and feel the signs and symptoms of distress, leave the office for a few minutes and walk up and down the stairs. This way you can avoid or reduce the symptoms of distress and will feel relaxed and ready to work productively. Staying in the office will only keep you in touch with the source of your distress.

Regular moderate exercise of 30 minutes a day changes the body's metabolism and helps maintain a desirable body weight. Exercise is an essential part of any slimming campaign. Furthermore, regular moderate exercise helps reduce the LDL-cholesterol ('bad' cholesterol) in the blood and increase HDL-cholesterol ('good' cholesterol) which is thought to give protection against heart disease.

Regular exercise leads to fitness. Feeling fit will increase your sense of well-being. You will feel good about yourself and therefore more able to face the demands and pressures of life. Exercise will also improve the quality of your sleep – another essential part of our coping resources.

Exercise need not be expensive. You do not have to rush out to buy the latest in sports fashion wear, or aids such as exercise bicycles and multigyms. Walking costs nothing and many other sports such as swimming and cycling are relatively inexpensive.

One important benefit of exercise and fitness activities is the possibility of increasing social contacts and developing new friendships at clubs or simply on an afternoon walk. Exercise and fitness should be fun and not a chore or too competitive. You will need to find an exercise that suits you – your abilities, schedules, personality. As a general rule choose an activity that would have been done in the days of your grandfather. For example, take up walking rather than squash, especially if you are unfit.

Do not rush into an exercise regime (Type As take note!), particularly if you are over 35 years old. Have a check-up with your doctor, particularly if you are an angina or heart attack sufferer, before you embark on an exercise programme. Always follow a programme which starts slowly and gradually increases to your prescribed level. Do not push yourself too hard. If you have any pains (particularly in your chest) or breathlessness, do not ignore them – stop at once and see your doctor as soon as possible. Better to be safe than sorry – exercise can kill!

Avoid exercising when you are unwell, particularly when suffering from flu and other infectious diseases, because infections can spread more easily to the heart muscle and this may lead to serious problems. Try not to exercise too soon after a

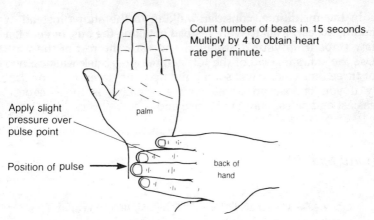

Count number of beats in 15 seconds.
Multiply by 4 to obtain heart
rate per minute.

Apply slight
pressure over
pulse point

palm

Position of pulse

back of
hand

Fig. 31   Measuring your pulse rate

meal. You should never exercise to the point where you do not have the breath to hold a conversation. Always keep a check on your heart rate by taking your pulse (Figure 31) and stay within the safe limits shown in the following table:

Maximum exercise pulse rate per minute

Age	Unfit person	Fit person
20	140	170
30	130	160
40	120	150
50	110	140
60	110	130
70	90	120

For an individual, these rates are only a general guide since there are many factors, such as general state of health, to take into account. You should consult your doctor before embarking on an exercise programme.

How do you decide on your level of fitness? A simple test is to check how fast your pulse returns to normal after you exercise. For fit people this usually occurs within a minute or two. If it takes a long time you are probably unfit. Electronic devices are available that can be worn by the user, thus giving an instant read-out of pulse rate (see page 201 for details).

In the meantime, consider walking to the shops instead of taking the car, walk to work instead of taking the bus, or get off a few stops from your destination and walk the rest of the way. Use the stairs instead of the lift. Ten minutes brisk walking two or three times a day will soon build up your stamina, particularly if you choose an uphill course. Walking is the cheapest, easiest and safest way to exercise and achieve fitness.

Body weight

- AIM TO MAINTAIN YOUR IDEAL BODY WEIGHT
- BALANCE ENERGY CONSUMED WITH ENERGY EXPENDED

Being overweight (or obese) is unhealthy and can cause much distress. Obesity has been cited as a contributory factor in diabetes, heart and circulatory diseases. Obesity can lower self-esteem and cause emotional problems. But how overweight do you have to be to increase your risk of ill health? It seems that the risk grows with an increasing level of obesity. A slight degree of obesity carries a slight risk and excessive overweight carries a high risk.

Body weight depends on a number of factors so how do you know if you are at your ideal weight, overweight or underweight? Simply taking height and age is not an accurate method of assessing this. Instead a measurement called the body mass index (BMI) is used. It is easily calculated by using the following method.

Step 1   Take your weight in kilograms or convert your weight in pounds to kilograms by multiplying by 0.45.

Step 2   Take your height in metres or convert your height in inches to metres by multiplying by 0.025.

Step 3   Square your height in metres, that is, multiply height in metres by itself (height in metres multiplied by height in metres).

Step 4   Divide weight in kilograms by height in metres squared.

Example
Male, height 5ft 6ins or 66 inches. Weight 160 pounds.

Step 1   160 pounds × 0.45 = 72 kilograms
Step 2   66 inches × 0.025 = 1.65 metres
Step 3   1.65 × 1.65 = 2.72
Step 4   72 ÷ 2.72 = 26.47. This is the BMI.

The ideal BMI for men is around 23 (acceptable range 20.5 to 26) and around 21 for women (acceptable range 19–23). So for this man, his ideal weight should be 23 × height squared, that is 23 × 2.72 = 62.56 kilograms. To convert kilograms to pounds divide by 0.45. In this case it is 139 pounds so he is about 21 pounds overweight (160 − 139 = 21). A BMI of over 30 carries a real health risk.

There are many causes of weight problems. Overeating and lack of exercise are obvious causes, hormone imbalances another and distress a less obvious candidate. Often being overweight is not the problem itself but a result of an individual's emotional problems. Lack of stimulation, leading to distress, can prompt overeating in an attempt to relieve boredom. This may take the form of picking at food throughout the day or bingeing, usually with highly calorific convenience foods. The obvious answer to boredom is to find something to occupy the time and to provide a new challenge, such as taking up a hobby, joining a club or starting a project at home. Lifestyle should be reviewed to find out why boredom occurred in the first place. This should then be tackled.

Low self-esteem is often the cause of compulsive eating and drinking, resulting in obesity which pushes self-esteem down further. So improving self-esteem (see page 194) can help avoid weight problems.

There are many advantages of being around your ideal weight. It is easier to become and stay fit when you have less weight to carry about. You will feel good about your appearance and be comfortable with yourself. So no wonder slimming campaigns, methods and aids flourish. However, there is probably no other health issue more controversial than slimming. The only answer to successful weight loss and maintenance of an ideal body weight is to balance energy (calorie) input (energy from the food we eat) with energy output (energy expended during your daily activities).

To lose weight, you need to take in fewer calories than you

expend. This should not be attempted in a drastic way by crash-dieting. Weight loss should be gradual. Eat fewer calories and expend more energy a little at a time. Assuming that there are no medical problems this method is guaranteed to work and costs very little. You will need:

- to know the calorie content of different foods
- to know how many calories are expended in different activities
- to know the number of calories required for your normal body processes
- to plan meals and activities
- will-power to avoid tempting high calorific foods
- time and patience.

The calorie counting method of weight control

Energy expended (output)

Activity	Kilocalories per ½-hour	Activity	Kilocalories per ½-hour
Sleeping	35	Washing and dressing	100
Walking (casual)	100	Light domestic work	75
Sitting eating	75	Sitting (relaxed)	50
Sitting writing	55	Shopping	100
Golf	100	Tennis	175
Swimming	250	Squash	325
Walking uphill	175	Jogging	150
Gardening	150	Driving	70
Cycling	100	Lying, relaxing	40

Firstly calculate your approximate energy expenditure by noting the calories used up during your daily activities, then estimate your energy intake by calculating your calorie intake. Make a note of the difference: energy expended minus energy consumed. If you want to lose weight your aim is to expend more energy than you consume. For every 3500 kilocalories you expend more than you consume, you will lose one pound of body fat. So if you can expend 100 more kilocalories than you eat during one day, it will take nearly a month for you to lose one pound. By using 500 calories more than you take in each day, you will lose one pound each week.

From the charts you will see that expending an extra 500 kilocalories each day is equivalent to 2½ hours walking or 2½

ENERGY CONSUMED (INPUT)			
Food	*Approx kcal per average helping*	*Food*	*Approx kcal per average helping*
Butter and		1 egg fried	140
margarine	100	Milk, skimmed in	
1 egg boiled	80	tea or coffee	5
Milk, whole, in		All-Bran cereal	90
tea or coffee	10	1 digestive biscuit	65
Yoghurt, pot	150	1 jam doughnut	250
Cornflakes	100	Bread, med. slice	80
1 cream cracker	70	Bacon, fried	
Boiled rice	130	(3 rashers)	340
Chicken (roast)	150	Beef steak, grilled	350
Sausage (2 large)	280	Banana	50
Potato, boiled	100	Apple (eating)	30
jacket, incl. skin	80	Grapefruit	
chips	300	(fresh ½)	20
roast	140	Orange	40
Ice cream	100	Chocolate bar	250
Beer, per pint	180	Sugar,	
Tea, no milk		per teaspoon	30
or sugar	0	Coffee, black	0
Cheddar cheese	130	Fruit juice,	
Camembert	100	unsweetened	70

This is obviously just a selection of calorific values. A more extensive list can be found in the *Complete Guide to Calories*, published by Slimming Magazine.

hours cycling or 1 hour swimming. It is often easier to reduce the number of calories consumed; one chocolate bar is equivalent in energy to 1¼ hours of walking. If you are overweight and embark on an exercise programme, you can achieve fitness and weight loss at the same time!

Unless a great deal of trouble is taken weighing everything you eat and timing everything you do, it must be accepted that these calculations are only approximations. But crude though it may be, this technique generates an awareness of the principles behind body weight control and if practised sensibly will lead to effective weight loss.

Remember, we do not eat simply to ensure that we have enough nutrition to live; it is also one of the pleasures of life.

Plan your diet so it is not boring and when you eat out choose your meals sensibly. Eat little and often so that you do not get hungry or feel tempted to eat a high calorie snack. Eat grilled rather than fried foods. Eat plenty of fresh fruit and vegetables. Try raw carrot, it is tasty and filling. Cut down on fats, sweets, biscuits and cakes.

Sleep and rest

- GET ADEQUATE SLEEP AND REST
- SET YOURSELF A SLEEP ROUTINE

Sleep and rest are essential for survival, health, fitness and well-being. Your brain and body systems can work at a different level of activity, allowing your batteries to recharge ready to face another day of stimulation, threats, challenges and activity.

The quality of sleep appears to be more important than quantity but too much or too little sleep can lead to irritability and poor mental performance. How long should you sleep? This varies enormously from person to person. Most people sleep seven hours each night whilst some need nine and others only five. Frequently, worry about losing sleep produces more symptoms of lack of sleep than the sleep loss itself.

If you are experiencing regular sleep disturbance, do not worry that this could be leading to ill health or lack of ability to perform. Even if your sleep patterns are erratic, you get more sleep than you think you have; certainly enough to avoid unhealthy consequences and very poor performance. Your body is geared to make sure you get enough sleep, otherwise you would not survive.

Stress is one of the main causes of sleep disturbance; lying awake at night, trying to get to sleep, worrying about current problems or becoming anxious about future events. When you eventually get to sleep you wake feeling tired and find the worries and anxieties are still there. People who are depressed usually have little difficulty getting to sleep but they often wake early.

It is also important to get the right pattern of sleep. The kind of sleep called rapid eye movement (REM) sleep, which results in dreaming, is very necessary. Dreaming, even if you cannot remember the dream, is the body's way of sorting out information and problems and ensuring that the body and mind have a complete rest. Alcohol as well as tranquillisers and barbiturates all decrease the amount of REM sleep so after taking them, you may wake up feeling tired or depressed. If you have nightmares, this may be a sign of anxiety or depression. Recurring nightmares are a sign of distress. Meditation can reduce the anxiety associated with nightmares and can help eliminate them altogether.

If you have sleep difficulties then try the following:

- Set up a routine that will condition you to get to sleep. Unplug the television, put the milk bottles out, have a warm milk drink (it contains tryptophan which promotes sleep), clean your teeth and lastly try reading a short *pleasant* story in bed.
- Avoid taking naps during the day or evening.
- Sit up in bed and meditate for five minutes and then lie down.
- Before going to bed avoid caffeine, too much alcohol, a heavy meal, particularly foods high in fibre and fats.
- Make sure you get plenty of exercise during the day.
- Set yourself a routine sleeping time: go to bed at the same time each night and rise at the same time each day.
- If your mind is racing get up and move around, go to the kitchen and make yourself a warm milk drink. When you have calmed down return to bed and try to think of a pleasant scene where you feel secure. Try to picture it in your mind's eye and concentrate on it.

Sleep well.

11   Reducing Type A Behaviour to Increase Coping Resources

HOW TO GET FROM A TO B

- SLOW DOWN, DO NOT HURRY, WHY RACE THE CLOCK?
- TACKLE ONE TASK AT A TIME AND ENJOY IT
- LEARN TO OCCUPY YOUR TIME WHILST WAITING
- ORGANISE YOUR DAILY ACTIVITIES TO AVOID QUEUES
- ACCEPT THE MISTAKES AND TRIVIALITIES OF YOURSELF AND OTHERS
- AVOID GETTING ANGRY OVER THINGS YOU CAN DO NOTHING ABOUT
- AVOID CREATING UNNECESSARY DEADLINES AND CLUTTERING UP YOUR CALENDAR WITH APPOINTMENTS
- SMILE AND GIVE LOVE AND AFFECTION
- PRACTISE BEING A GOOD LISTENER
- LEARN TO RELAX; LOOK AROUND AND APPRECIATE NATURE AND YOUR ENVIRONMENT
- PLAY GAMES FOR FUN AND NOT SIMPLY TO WIN

Type A s, through their beliefs, attitudes and habits, frequently perceive situations as threatening and challenging when no real threat or challenge exists. A traffic jam or a slow-moving supermarket queue is clearly not life-threatening but they can provoke anger which activates the aggressive fight part of the alarm reaction.

How does Type A behaviour arise? Studies of the prevalence of Type A behaviour in identical and fraternal twins have shown that Type A is not inherited although some of its component behaviours, such as aggression and hostility, may be genetically determined. Other studies have shown that Type A behaviour is learnt. Type A children, particularly boys, tend to have Type A parents. Researchers have shown that one of the ways in which children learn to behave in a Type A manner is by copying their parents.

A child's upbringing can result in Type A behaviour being manifested from an early age. If parents fail to provide unconditional love (love without pre-conditions) or set never-ending standards and expectations, then the child's self-worth and self-esteem diminishes. At school the child seizes any opportunity to perform well to boost their low self-esteem. Soon, self-worth and self-esteem become measured by achievements, particularly where it is believed these are admired by parents and others. The struggle to achieve and to secure control over their environment continues into adult life, especially in their attempt to climb the career ladder. In doing so the individual has learned to behave in a way that can be self-destructive in the long run.

So if Type A behaviour is learned then it can be 'unlearned'. Recent research has shown that Type A behaviour can be modified and reduced. In one study, the Recurrent Coronary Prevention Project (RCPP), over a thousand men and women who had already had one heart attack were recruited for a programme designed to modify their Type A behaviour. The study set out to discover whether Type A behaviour can be modified and whether such modification alters the risk of having a second heart attack. The recruits were divided into three main groups. Group 1 received the usual advice on what to do following a heart attack; for example, advice on diet, exercise and so on. Group 2 were given the same advice but also underwent a programme of Type A behaviour modification. Group 3 was a control group; they received no treatment at all.

The Type A behaviour modification counselling programme ran for one year and the fate of all the recruits in the study was followed in the succeeding 3½ years. The results showed that Type A behaviour can be modified and reduced. Furthermore, those in Group 2 who significantly changed their Type A behaviour reduced by half their chance of suffering a second heart attack (both fatal and non-fatal) compared to those in either of the other groups.

Another study by the same researchers demonstrated that Type A behaviour can be modified in healthy individuals, thus indicating that Type As do not have to be ill to have the motivation to change their behaviour.

In both these studies the Type A behaviour reduction was accompanied by a decrease in blood cholesterol levels, suggesting that the participants were generating less stress for themselves and therefore less catecholamines. Furthermore, those who changed their Type A behaviour became calmer and more in control of situations. They improved their self-esteem and sense of well-being. They became better listeners. They stopped trying to do too many things at once, so they could pay better attention to the particular task in hand. They were more pleasant to be with. Almost without exception they found that changes in their behaviour not only improved their family and social relationships but actually enhanced their careers!

So the popular image of a Type A individual who is ambitious, highly competitive, aggressive, hard-driving, a high achiever and therefore highly successful is not altogether true. The more relaxed, calmer, unhurried but still ambitious Type B individual proves to be just as successful, or more so, in the long run. The difference is that Type Bs achieve the same goals but without paying the price of ill health. Many companies have seen the benefits of Type A behaviour modification. They have arranged Type A behaviour treatment for their employees, recognising that it improves their work efficiency and productivity as well as maintaining health. This clearly adds up to a substantial financial saving.

Most of us display some degree of Type A behaviour so we can all benefit from taking a more Type B approach to life. Reduction of your Type A behaviour can be achieved only by examining your beliefs, attitudes and habits; those habits with which you have burdened your life. A chronic sense of time urgency or a tendency to become easily upset and angry over trivia must be discarded or modified. To do this you must substitute new, healthy beliefs for your bad, unhealthy ones. The RCPP objective for treating Type A behaviour was to change Anger, Irritation, Aggravation and Impatience (AIAI) into Acceptance (of the errors yourself and of others), Serenity, Affection and Self-esteem enhancement (ASAS).

AIAI to ASAS

There are a number of ways of tackling this and they all take time to learn and practise; there is no quick way to unlearn or modify what has taken years to learn.

Drilling

As a start, set yourself drills aimed to make you do the opposite to what you normally do. For example, if you get impatient whilst waiting then your drill would be to find a queue and practise waiting without getting impatient. Keep with you a paperback to read or a pack of postcards to write to friends or to make notes or plans for a DIY project. You might say avoiding queues is the best answer. Yes but, being realistic, you cannot get through life these days without queueing at some time or another. If you travel by car you will almost certainly get caught in traffic jams. In this case take the opportunity to relax; put the gear in neutral, handbrake on, feet on the floor, breathe deeply and slowly, and recall a pleasant memory.

Review your driving habits – do you drive fast? Race the red light? Do a Grand Prix start on green? Overtake and weave in and out of traffic? If so, then set yourself drills such as driving mainly in the slow lane and keeping to one lane.

Make a list of your Type A behaviours using the description of Type A we provided earlier (see page 102) then make a diary of drills appropriate for your treatment. For example:

Monday:	Speak more slowly.
Tuesday:	Tackle one task/thing at a time (instead of polyphasing).
Wednesday:	Keep mainly in the left-hand traffic lane (instead of weaving from one lane to another to get in the fastest moving lane).
Thursday:	Walk more slowly.
Friday:	Linger at the table (instead of rushing away as soon as you finish eating).
Saturday:	Seek a long queue and practise waiting patiently (instead of getting impatient and irritated).
Sunday:	Leave your watch off and practise being less time urgent (instead of letting time dictate your day).

Each day, concentrate on the specified drill. So for Monday, concentrate on speaking more slowly; for Tuesday do only one task at a time, and so on. Gradually, with regular drilling, you will replace your old Type A behaviours with new Type B behaviours. After a while these will become a habit in just the same way as you learned your Type A behaviours which formed your old habits. Without noticing, you will soon be practising Type B behaviours each day of the week and not only on your specified drill day.

Accept that your change from Type A towards Type B will take a long time to achieve. You will find it useful to construct a drill diary for each day of the year. Here is a list of suggested drills to assign randomly to each day of the year. You will need to use each one several times along with your own drills.

DRILLS

- Walk more slowly
- Speak more slowly
- Say . . . 'Maybe I'm wrong'
- Leave your watch off
- Listen to music for 15 minutes
- Linger at the table after a meal
- Recall pleasant memories for 10 minutes
- Buy a small gift for a friend, partner or family member
- Drive in the slow lane
- Practise listening during conversations
- Notice objects around you: trees, flowers
- Practise eradicating hostile grimaces
- Stop fist clenches and knee jiggles
- Verbalise affection for your partner and children
- Observe facial expression (your own and others)
- Ask a friend about themselves
- Set aside 30 minutes for yourself
- Eat more slowly
- Practise smiling
- Practise assertiveness
- Seek a long queue
- Read for 30 minutes
- Alter one of your usual habits or ways of doing things
- Substitute understanding for anger
- Soak in a bath for 15 minutes
- Practise anger control
- Visit a museum, art gallery or park
- Contact an old friend – someone with a job or profession different from yours
- Refer to yourself less often in conversations

These drills are aimed at alleviating your sense of time urgency and easily aroused anger and hostility.

Cueing

To help you modify your Type A behaviour we have included with this book a strip of self-adhesive red hearts which remind you to practise your drills. Place one in the centre of your watch glass as a reminder to rid yourself of your chronic sense of time urgency. Every time you glance at your watch remember your drills. Place a heart on your steering wheel or dashboard as a reminder to rid yourself of Type A driving habits. Place one on the telephone to act as a cue to tackle one task at a time and not to polyphase whilst speaking. How about one on your placemat at the dinner table reminding you to eat more slowly and to linger at the table?

Your heart clip can be used as a cue in your diary. It will remind you to slow down, not to clutter your day with appointments, to avoid creating unnecessary deadlines and to leave some time in the day for yourself.

We deliberately use hearts as cueing devices because of the association between Type A behaviour and the heart. Many participants in our stress management programmes find that this association, together with their awareness of the stress response and Type A behaviour, motivates them more than anything else to modify their behaviour. As a typical example of this, a man related to us his experience whilst driving at the start of his counselling programme. 'I was sitting in the traffic jam staying in the slow lane but I could feel my noradrenaline start to flow. I looked at the heart on the steering wheel and reminded myself that the way I was feeling could allow noradrenaline to strike at my heart. A traffic jam is not worth dying for so I turned my cassette on, sat back and relaxed. It was interesting watching those ignorant of this fact gambling with their life in more ways than one!'

Monitoring

Regular drilling takes a great deal of will-power. You will find it helpful to ask your family and friends to act as monitors. Explain to them what you are doing and ask them to monitor your progress. They can remind you to drill if you lapse into your old Type A ways. The wife of a man on our programme hummed the television show 'A Team' theme tune each time her husband lapsed into his Type A ways. Your monitors may also suggest drills for Type A behaviours you are unaware you possess; Type As are often blind to their own behaviour. Ask your monitors to read the section on Type A behaviour and invite their comments on the way you behave. Be prepared to listen carefully to your monitors' observations. They can provide you with support and at the same time help themselves to modify their own Type A behaviour.

Examining your beliefs

Alleviating your sense of time urgency and managing your time effectively

Question your Type A time urgent belief. Answer true or false to this statement; *'Being time urgent has helped me gain success'*.

If you answer 'true', then think carefully. How successful are you? It may be that any failures are a result of mistakes that could have been avoided if you had been patient and taken time to think and organise, to be creative and innovative. For this reason, some drills are designed to rid you of your haste; for example, eat, talk, walk, drive more slowly and avoid polyphasing.

Ask yourself if frantically switching traffic lanes gets you to work quicker. Carry on driving in your usual manner for the next week and time your journey each day. Then the following week keep in one lane (where this is possible) and time your journeys. Now take the average journey time for each week. Most drivers find a difference in their journey time of only a few minutes. Now think; is it worth exposing your heart to potentially fatal levels of noradrenaline to save a few minutes each day?

Other drills are aimed to repair damage done by years of time urgency. Type As have little time to recall memories, so some time should be allocated to this activity. Review your life and plan ahead, setting realistic goals.

Years of struggling to do more and more in less time encourages the Type A individual to concentrate on achievements and strategies to gain or maintain control. There is little space in their lives for relaxation or cultural activities. To correct this, stop measuring your life in quantities; number of committees served on, amount of money earned, number of accomplishments, etc. Think instead in terms of quality of life. To help bring this about, your diary should include drills such as reading more (but not technical, financial or material associated with your job), visiting museums, art galleries, theatres and observing nature.

'One ought, every day at least, to hear a little song, read a good poem, see a fine picture and if it were possible, to speak a few reasonable words.'   Goethe

When we asked the wife of one of our Type A group participants if she had noticed any change in her husband's behaviour, she said, 'Whilst we were driving in Wales, Peter commented on the beauty of the scenery. He never did this before the course. It may sound a small thing but when you spend all your time rushing from A to B a change like this is noticeable.' Remember how, in the Prologue, Frank said he now sees more of life and in particular more of the countryside? These are just two examples of taking time for living. Try taking off your watch; you will find that you have all the time in the world. Take time to look around to see what pleasurable things can be found. You will then rid yourself of your obsession with numbers and quantities and instead describe in words the beauty of things surrounding you.

Ask yourself: are you preoccupied with your own attempts to achieve your goals? Workaholics are blind to the fact that they are not giving time to their families. Even major events in the lives of their children go unnoticed. A recent survey of workaholics revealed some disturbing and sad indicators of this exclusive preoccupation with self and ambitions. A small child drew a picture of his family; Mummy, sister and himself – but Daddy was missing. Another child waiting for his father at the airport was reported to have asked several men, 'Are you my Daddy?' How often we have heard our reformed Type As sadly express regret at missing much of their children's development. The missed school sports, parents' evenings, nativity plays and so on. Once gone they cannot be replaced.

Review your activities to make time for the things that are important. Winston Churchill said, 'When a man cannot distinguish a great from a small event, he is of no use.'

Learn how to manage your time effectively. Our lives are dominated by time and for Type As, time is more of a problem than others. We all know there are 24 hours in each day and we like to use our waking hours effectively. Nobody likes wasting time unnecessarily: it is in reality losing part of one's life. But if you become obsessed with time the resultant distress could be shortening your life and certainly reducing its quality.

Managing your time effectively at work is important if you wish to avoid distress. The section on reducing demands suggested a number of ways in which you can do this by planning, prioritising, setting realistic goals, being assertive, avoiding perfectionism, saying no and delegating. You will also be more time-effective if you tackle jobs which require mental effort when you feel at your best and able to concentrate; in other words when you are in the eustress zone. Do the tasks requiring less mental effort when you are not able to concentrate as well or when you anticipate interruptions. Do not waste time worrying unnecessarily about future events. Remember, *it's not the hours you put in – it's what you put into the hours that counts*.

Balancing your time between family, leisure, work and sleep is important. Regularly spending long periods at work will inevitably mean less time for your family and for leisure activities. Too much work often leads to mental fatigue and difficulty in relaxing, which will inevitably affect the quality of the time spent with your family and friends. Finding time to spend with your partner, children, family and friends will enable you to nurture love and support and to enhance your self-esteem and happiness.

Include in your daily schedule periods for relaxation, exercise and time for you to spend on your own. Pamper yourself each day. Build 'idling time' into your routine so as not to rush the things you do. Allow plenty of time for washing, dressing and eating breakfast even if it means rising half-an-hour earlier in the morning. Spend time on meditation and muscular relaxation. Allow more time than you estimate for journeys and give yourself time to be punctual for appointments. In this way, you will reduce anxiety if you are unexpectedly delayed.

Remember, there are 168 hours in each week so there is time to devote to everything, so sit down and plan how you want to spend your time. Time is precious and we all want to spend it happily. So remember, for every sixty seconds you are angry you lose a minute of happiness.

Alleviating your easily aroused anger and hostility

Question your Type A anger and hostility beliefs. Answer true or false to this statement; *'I need aggression and hostility to succeed'*.

If your answer is 'true', then consider that by using aggression and hostility rather than understanding, you may damage your health and your relationships with family, friends and work colleagues. In the long run, this will not lead to success.

Making mistakes, failing to achieve goals, receiving adverse criticism, particularly in front of others, and perceiving a situation as unfair or embarrassing can trigger frustration and anger. As we described earlier such emotion leads to excessive release of noradrenaline, the potential killer. When you next feel yourself getting irritated, aggravated and angry remember that, if triggered, your anger can inflict the most damage on the person you least intend – yourself. Train yourself to avoid anger: do not get hooked, practise anger control and use the quieting reflex (p. 142).

Try these two techniques; avoiding the hook and anger control.

Avoiding the hook

Picture yourself as a fish in a river. Every morning you wake up and start swimming. The waters ahead appear clear but on the banks of the river are anglers casting their hooks, hoping to catch you. Suddenly a worm on a hook appears in front of you. The bait looks tempting but if you bite you will be hooked. Think; 'Bite or pass by?'. You pass by, avoiding the bait. Unexpectedly another hook drops in front of you. Ask yourself; 'Bite or pass by?'. You pass by, only to find more hooks appearing along your journey.

Type As bite all the time, perhaps thirty to forty times a day. The problem is that we have no idea when the next hook is going to appear and this makes anger and hostility difficult to deal with.

Anger control

If you feel yourself starting to take the bait, then say 'stop'. Detach yourself from the situation and analyse your behaviour and feelings. Ask yourself, 'What provoked me?'. Identify the causes of your anger and the beliefs, attitudes and feelings that led you to take the bait. Now replay the situation again in your mind to see whether the way in which you acted was appropriate, justified and rational. Usually you will find taking the bait serves no real purpose. Remain calm and hold a conversation with yourself (called **self-talk**); 'It's not worth getting worked up about', 'There is no real reason to argue', 'Keep cool, don't take the bait', 'Unpleasantness can lead to more unpleasantness', 'Practise QR', 'Reason it out'.

The trick is not to take the bait and therefore not to get angry in the first place. Do not get hooked on things you cannot do anything about. So if the train is delayed and you are late for your appointment, use self-talk to accept that there is nothing you can do to make up the lost time. Instead use your energy to think about alleviating the problem. When you arrive at the station, telephone your appointment, explain the situation and say you will be arriving as soon as possible. You also have little control over the errors and antics of others, so learn to accept their mistakes and trivialities. If you cannot, this will inevitably lead to frustration, anger and hostility.

Work at lessening your sense of time urgency. Impatience is a mild form of irritation which in turn is a mild form of anger. Above all, recognise that your anger and hostility are manifestations of your low self-esteem. When self-esteem is high then anger, aggression and hostility will be low. Blows to your self-esteem will easily trigger hostility, so work toward enhancing your self-esteem and practise being assertive. Note that your self-esteem is affected by the degree of love and affection in your life so when love and affection are present self-esteem will be high and the potential for hostility will be low. Learning to give and receive love and affection is therefore vital in your battle against anger and hostility. Tell your partner and children how much you value their love, affection and support and express your feelings to them. Take an interest in your friends and share their ups and downs. Also learn to laugh at yourself and your mistakes and errors. Stop taking yourself too seriously!

For once, it is better to be in the 'B' team rather than the 'A' team.

12 Improving Personal Life Skills to Increase Coping Resources

- INCREASE LOVE AND SUPPORT
- ENHANCE SELF-ESTEEM
- LEARN TO BE ASSERTIVE
- THINK POSITIVELY
- SMILE
- LAUGH
- DEVELOP A SENSE OF HUMOUR

Increasing love and support

The importance of love and support in helping you deal with distress cannot be emphasised strongly enough. A considerable amount of research has shown that those people with low love and social support succumb to health problems more easily than those with high levels of love and support. It is easy to see why if we remember the effects of stress hormones. When a person feels secure, loved and well supported, noradrenaline, adrenaline and cortisol levels are all lower than normal.

In discussing love and support, we intend this to be interpreted in its broadest sense. This includes not only our intimate relationships but also affection and respect between friends and support at work from colleagues.

Within the family

Love and support within the family is naturally our first experience. The parent-child relationship is crucial in moulding the future life of the child. Time and time again I (TL) see people in my private consultancy who have memories of being unloved during their childhood, of conflict with parents and jealousy of the affection and love given to brothers and sisters but not to them. Many times I have heard, 'My mother (or father) didn't love me'. The result sitting in front of me is a very depressed person with a variety of psychological problems, and usually a bottle of tranquillisers.

Love is one of our basic needs. From the cradle we yearn to be cuddled, hugged and kissed particularly when we face the pressures and demands of growing up. Lack of love and affection or feeling unwanted often leads to problems in later life particularly when it comes to courtship, sexual relationships and parenting.

In adulthood touching, stroking and caressing are essential in developing relationships. Under the right circumstances this is undoubtedly the best way to relax, reduce tension and therefore reduce distress. The direct power of this on our health is difficult to investigate but stroking has been shown to be extremely therapeutic and has great impact on our well-being and health.

Those living alone but with a pet have been shown to have lower blood pressure, a lower incidence of sudden cardiac death and quicker recovery rates following operations than non-pet owners who live alone. Lonely heart attack victims with pets tend to live longer than those who do not own a pet. Having a pet provides the opportunity for stroking, and a sense of belonging and not feeling isolated.

An experiment designed to investigate dietary fat intake and arterial disease in rabbits unexpectedly provided a good illustration of the powers of touching, stroking and affection. The researchers found that although all rabbits in the experiment were fed the same high-fat diet and lived in the same conditions, a small number failed to develop significant arterial disease. No reason could be found until it was realised that this particular group of rabbits was cared for by a technician who regularly stroked and cuddled each rabbit. Rabbits not receiving this treatment all developed significant arterial disease. So amazed were the researchers when they realised that cuddling and stroking might have this effect that they set up an experiment to test it. They repeated the original experiment but this time deliberately included the cuddling and stroking in one group of rabbits. The result was the same as in the first experiment. Those animals receiving physical attention developed very little coronary heart disease.

So do not underestimate the power and benefits of touching and caressing. Express your love and affection to your partner, children and family. Cuddle your partner or children whilst watching television (this is good polyphasing!). Respond to their signals of 'I want to be cuddled'. Too often the demands and pressures of work and parenting turn what were the exciting honeymoon years of marriage into a dreary relationship. When did you last say to your spouse, 'I love you'? When did you last buy your partner a small gift? Rekindle the courting years; ask your partner out to dinner next weekend and treat the occasion as your first date. Purchase a small gift for your partner, children or parents, or take your family out for a treat. Spend more time with them; so often we hear people's sadness and regrets over the lack of time given to their children.

In friendships

The value of friendships is incalculable. It is not necessarily the number of friends you have that counts but the quality of the friendships. One true friend is worth far more than several acquaintances. True friends share one another's interests and successes as well as failures. With a true friend you can express yourself and be accepted for what and who you are. At work, mutual support between colleagues can be of tremendous help in getting the job done and reducing distress for everyone.

Sharing problems

Family and friends should be people with whom you can share your problems, to seek advice and sympathy. Undoubtedly one of the key values of love and support is being able to share and talk over problems with someone else. As the saying goes, 'A trouble shared is a trouble halved'. Talk over your problems at home and work, and help others by listening. Do not bottle things up inside; talk ..., talk ..., talk ..., express your feelings to whomever you feel most comfortable and confident with.

Enhancing self-esteem

Self-esteem is the self-evaluation we make of our worth as a person. It is based on how competent, significant, likeable and successful we think we are. Feeling good about ourselves (high self-esteem) reduces distress and provides the platform for eustress, personal growth and development, effectiveness and creativity.

Our self-esteem is based largely on the relationship between our actual achievements and what we want and expect out of life. When achievements exceed expectations then self-esteem rises. On the other hand, failure to achieve expectations results in low self-esteem. This is where Type As find most of their problems; they set themselves never-ending and unrealistic targets and goals which they rarely achieve. As a result, they struggle to secure adequate self-esteem. Since Type As believe that self-esteem can be enhanced only by achieving, they set themselves yet more unattainable targets and goals. Failure is usually more frequent than success, so self-esteem is further lowered. A vicious circle is established.

When self-esteem is low the potential for anger and hostility is high. So when Type As fail to achieve their expectations, their self-esteem is lowered and they become frustrated, irritable, angry and hostile. Aggression is then used in an attempt to achieve the impossible.

Type Bs, on the other hand, have much more realistic expectations. As a result, their achievements often surpass their expectations so self-esteem is rarely dented and remains secure.

One of the most difficult things in life is to discover yourself and to set yourself realistic goals and expectations which you feel able to achieve. You may need to be content with achieving less than 100%.

Praise and recognition for a job well done is guaranteed to raise self-esteem. This is a good management strategy for establishing and maintaining a happy and productive work-force. With self-esteem high, co-operation is more likely. When dealing with others, remember that their self-esteem is easily damaged by adverse criticism of their work, mistakes and shortcomings. Also, praise yourself for a task well done by using self-talk.

Changing your self-image (how you see yourself) means reviewing all aspects of your life. Accept your faults and insecurities and work to resolve them. Harness your strengths and capitalise on them. Do not try to be what you feel others want you to be, be honest with yourself and others, express yourself; grow beyond what you are.

Looking good, feeling healthy, fit and loved, smiling, develop-ing a sense of humour, not taking life or yourself too seriously and being assertive are all self-esteem boosters.

Thinking positively

Think positively. You will gain more from life by thinking positively than by taking a cautious and negative approach. In other words, be an optimist rather than a pessimist. This will help reduce anxiety since pessimists often live with the fear of failure. For each situation you meet, you can be negative or positive. Look to the positive aspects and learn and gain something from everything you do. When things go wrong, learn from your mistakes and do not dwell on your failures. Each time you find yourself thinking negatively switch to positive thinking by using self-talk: 'It can't be this bad – there must be something I can gain from this situation'. One of the fuels for negative thinking is unnecessary worry about future events, particularly when you are not in possession of the full facts, so avoid uncertainty.

Learning to be assertive

Being assertive is a most effective way of increasing your coping resources. Assertiveness is simply a way of communicating effectively. It means being able to say what you feel, think or want. It also means being able to understand other people's points of view and to negotiate and reach a workable compromise in awkward situations. Behaving assertively will boost your self-esteem and reduce anger and aggression.

We are all assertive to some degree. However, we can learn to be more effective communicators. Here is an example of assertiveness.

A work colleague asks to borrow your book. You know this person has a reputation for never returning borrowed material. Your assertive response might be,

'I realise that you need material from this book'.

This lets the other person know that you heard and understood their request. You then say,

'However, I do not like to lend my books'.

This states how you feel or what you think. You finally add,

'I suggest that you try the library, I know they have a copy'.

By this statement, you are making some recommendations. You let the other person know that you want to help by making constructive suggestions.

Your first statement, *'I realise that you need material from this book'*, tells the other person that you acknowledge what is being said and that you understand what they are saying. This statement should begin with a phrase such as 'I understand' or 'I realise' or 'I appreciate'. When you get into the habit of using this approach you will find yourself listening to (not just hearing) what someone is saying. This is a good drill for modifying Type A behaviour.

Your second statement should always start with the word 'However'. NEVER say 'but' because this is an aggressive word. Now you need to express your feelings about this issue. State clearly what you feel or think . . . *'I do not like to lend my books'*. You have to be honest with yourself and this takes courage. Everyone has a right to say how they feel. By being honest you will feel better afterwards. This will also help raise your self-esteem and increase self-respect and self-confidence. There is no suppression or bottling-up of emotions so the potential for activating your stress response is decreased and there is less chance of hostility. Again, a good drill for reducing Type A behaviour and learning to say 'no'.

The third statement, *'I suggest that you try the library, I know they have a copy'*, should be a constructive suggestion on what to do about the situation. You must state what you want or what action you want taken. It is important to be positive here and this may lead to negotiating and arriving at a workable compromise. Starting this statement with one of the following phrases is useful: 'I'd prefer it if . . .', 'I suggest that . . .', 'I'd appreciate it if . . .', and so on. It is important not to become aggressive here – do not tell the other person to get lost or words to that effect. You must provide them with a constructive suggestion.

Notice that the above example illustrates a reasonable, rational answer. This is what being assertive is all about – being reasonable. If you are reasonable then the other person is less likely to take offence. You have shown this person that you appreciate what is being asked, you have explained how you feel about the matter and you have been helpful. In other words, you have not been aggressive, you have not been passive – you have been assertive! Communication has been effective, progress has been made, you have responded in a Type B manner and you have handled the situation appropriately with no distress to yourself.

What if the other person becomes insistent or aggressive about your assertive response? In this case, you simply repeat your previous comments, keeping to the three steps: understand . . ., however . . ., and suggest . . . This way you will eventually arrive at a workable solution. With practice you will gain confidence in being assertive and this will take much of the distress out of life.

On some occasions, you may find that being assertive does not do the trick. It may be that a source of conflict remains unresolved no matter how assertive you are. It is important not to become too upset about this and not to blame yourself or others, otherwise your confidence will be undermined. Instead, try to look upon the situation positively and use self-talk, as described in the section on anger control. When you find that, by being assertive, you have solved a problem successfully, then congratulate yourself by self-talk. Praising yourself in this way will also show you the value of praising others.

Smiling and laughing and developing a sense of humour

It may be a strange thing to say, but many people appear to have lost the ability to smile. Just look around you to see what we mean. A genuine facial smile should reflect a 'smile' from your heart. Seeing someone smile will usually make you smile. Smiling makes you feel happy.

This is probably because smiling relaxes many of the facial muscles, thereby improving blood flow to the brain. More facial muscles are used for frowning and in anger than when smiling. Look in the mirror, screw your face up in angry grimaces and look at how many muscles you are using. Now smile. You will see that far fewer muscles are used as you smile.

Learn to avoid going about your daily activities with a worried or angry look on your face. Smile instead; you not only feel better but others relate to you more easily. So start the day with a 'heartfelt' smile. Smiling is a good way of coping with stress and reducing irritation, anger and hostility. Joking and laughter can defuse tense and awkward situations.

The British Safety Council recognises the benefits of smiling and laughter in reducing accident proneness and in improving work performance. They actually hold a 'Smile for Safety' week. A recent study has shown that humour at work eases mental tension, aids concentration and enhances creativity. No wonder some companies now hold humour workshops for their employees.

Laughter and humour can have a powerful effect on the mind and body. The story of Norman Cousins illustrates this point. Almost crippled by an incurable disease, he decided to take his treatment into his own hands. He read humorous books, jokes and watched comedy films. After a short time he recovered sufficiently to return to work. Norman put his recovery down to 'laughter therapy'. At the time there was much scepticism about his claim but today many researchers and doctors believe that laughter can induce changes in body activity that improve the circulation and digestion and reduce muscle tension. In fact, many of the effects are the opposite to those seen in distress. So perhaps we should include laughing sessions in our daily routine.

It is important that we learn to laugh at ourselves. Widows of heart attack victims often report that their husbands had lost their sense of humour and the ability to laugh at themselves. People who have a sense of humour have learnt to laugh at themselves and not to take life too seriously. In fact, a sense of humour is high on the list of what we look for in other people when forming relationships.

No wonder it is said that laughter is the best medicine.

Stresswise

Products and services available from Stresswise

Courses and consultancy

Stresswise: stress awareness and stress management programmes presented by Dr Terry Looker and Dr Olga Gregson.

Workshops and seminars are held regularly at centres throughout the country for industry, commerce and the professions. Programmes for the general public are held in Manchester, London, Norwich, Bristol and Edinburgh. For companies, programmes are offered 'in-house' or at venues throughout the United Kingdom.

Enquiries: Dr Terry Looker/Dr Olga Gregson, Department of Biological Sciences, John Dalton Building, Manchester Polytechnic, Manchester M1 5GD.

Biodots, self-adhesive red hearts and Stresswise heart clips

Available in small quantities and bulk purchase.

Stresswise relaxation tape

15 minute audio tape of progressive (side 1) and deep (side 2) muscular relaxation.

Galvanic skin response monitor and relaxation kit

Including biofeedback audio tape and information booklet.

Pulse/heart rate meters

Including digital quartz wristwatch; multifunctional, including heart rate monitor.

Personal fitness, nutritional and stress assessments

3 programmes developed by CALM (Computer Assisted Lifestyle Management) designed to assess your lifestyle and provide recommendations and suggestions for positive changes. You simply answer a questionnaire, which is then analysed and a personalised report prepared.

For price list and further details, send stamped addressed envelope to *Stresswise*, PO Box 5, Congleton, Cheshire CW12 1XE. State product(s) required.

Further Reading

Treating Type A behavior and your heart, Dr Meyer Friedman and Diane Ulmer. (Alfred A. Knopf, 1984)

Type A behavior and your heart, Dr Meyer Friedman and Dr Ray Rosenman. (Wildwood House Ltd/Fawcett, 1974)

Understanding stress, how to recognise the causes and effects of stress and what steps to take to come to terms with them.

(Consumers Association/Hodder and Stoughton, 1988)
(Includes chapters on stress in marriage, childhood and divorce, work stress, discussion of relaxation techniques)

The BUPA manual of fitness and well-being. (MacDonald Books, 1984)

The good health kit, a complete interactive fitness programme, Dr Richard Smith and Ron Van Der Meer. (Ebury Press, 1987)
(Contains tips on choosing a healthy diet, calorie guide, weight control, fitness and exercise guide)

Fighting heart disease, a practical self-help guide to prevention and treatment, Dr Chandra Patel. (Dorling Kindersley, 1987)
(Contains useful chapters on healthy eating, reducing alcohol consumption, giving up smoking, relaxation exercises and keeping fit as well as a clear and informative account of the heart and disease (angina and heart attacks))

How to survive the 9–5, Martin Lucas, Kim Wilson and Emma Hart. (Thames Methuen, 1986)
(Deals with occupational stress)

Stress, diet and your heart, Dr Dean Ornish. (Holt Rinehart and Winston, 1982)
(A supplement to the conventional medical treatment of coronary heart disease with chapters on stress management techniques and diet)

Assertiveness at work, a practical guide to handling awkward situations, K and K Back. (McGraw-Hill, 1982)

Getting things done, a radical new approach to managing time and achieving more at work, Roger Black. (Michael Joseph, 1987)

Don't do, delegate, the secret power of successful managers, James M Jenks and John M Kelly. (Kogan Page, 1986)

Smile therapy, how smiling and laughter can change your life, Liz Hodgkinson. (Macdonald Optima, 1987)

The book of massage, the complete step-by-step guide to Eastern and Western techniques, Lucinda Lidell. (Ebury Press, 1984)

Dr Vernon Coleman's guide to alternative medicine, a critical look at alternative medicine from the patient's point of view, Dr Vernon Coleman. (Corgi Books, 1988)

Complete guide to calories, a *Slimming* magazine publication, available from newsagents.